EVIDENCE BASED DIET

A PICTORIAL REPRESENTATION OF NUTRITION FACTS TO HELP YOU STAY HEALTHY.

VILLE KAAJAKARI, PhD

Evidence Based Diet.

ISBN: 978-0-9822991-8-0
Designed by Jennifer Smith

CONTENTS

PROLOGUE 6

INTRODUCTION 8

Nutritional science 10

Book outline 12

Disclaimer 13

PART 1 .... **14**

HEART DISEASE **17**

High cholesterol increases the risk of heart disease 18

Optimal LDL cholesterol is 50-70 mg/dL 19

Apolipoprotein may be a superior indicator of cardiovascular risks compared to standard cholesterol measurement 20

Heart disease risk factors dramatically affect life expectancy 22

Diabetes increases cardiovascular mortality 24

Vegetarian diet lowers cholesterol 25

Affluent diet raises cholesterol in one week 26

Cholesterol level for Indigenous People is below 150 mg/dL 27

High glycemic index foods increase heart disease risk 30

Fruit and vegetables protect from heart disease 32

Oat bran lower cholesterol 33

Whole grain decrease heart disease risk 34

Trans fats increase heart disease risk 35

Trans fats occur naturally in animal products 36

Milk fat increases heart disease mortality 37

Saturated fat increases cholesterol levels 38

Replacing saturated fats decreases heart disease risk 39

Unsaturated fats decrease the risk of heart disease 40

Omega-6/Omega-3 ratio may be important for heart health 41

Homocysteine is toxic to heart 43

Optimal B12 level is achieved with fortified foods or supplements 44

Nuts lower cholesterol 46

Nuts can cut heart disease risk in half 47

Red meat increases risk of death from heart disease 48

Low carb/high protein diets increase heart disease risk 49

A meal with saturated fat dramatically affects blood vessels 50

Vascular activity drops after eating fast food . . . 51
High-salt meals impair blood vessels . . . 52
Vinegar may improve cholesterol . . . 53
Calorie restriction improves heart health markers . . . 54
Alternate day fasting lowers cholesterol . . . 55
Vitamin D deficiency increases risk of death from heart disease . . . 56
Proper hydration can reduce the risk of death from heart disease . . . 57
Erectile dysfunction may be due to heart disease . . . 58
Coffee can raise cholesterol . . . 59
Key takeaways on heart disease . . . 60

DIABETES . . . 62
24-hour insulin profile is elevated for obese people . . . 64
Type-2 diabetes is low on plant-based diets . . . 66
Saturated fats decrease insulin sensitivity . . . 68
Elevated fasting glucose increases diabetes risk . . . 69
Elevated hemoglobin A1c increases diabetes risk . . . 70
High glycemic index foods increase diabetes risk . . . 71
Insulin index may be a better way to rank foods than glycemic index . . . 72
Berries moderate blood glucose . . . 74
Eating berries lowers type-2 diabetes risk . . . 75
Eating nuts lowers type-2 diabetes risk . . . 76
Eating fruits and vegetables lowers type-2 diabetes risk . . . 77
Meat increases diabetes risk . . . 78
Insulin response increases with combination of sugar + beef . . . 79
Insulin response is spiked by milk . . . 80
Vinegar improves glucose and insulin response . . . 81
Lowering body mass index (BMI) improves fasting glucose . . . 82
Fasting lowers insulin levels . . . 83
Key takeaways on diabetes . . . 84

CANCER **86**

Diet and obesity cause most cancers. 87

Meat consumption increases cancer risk 88

Alcohol increases cancer risk 90

Low body mass index (BMI) minimizes cancer risk. 91

High glycemic index diet increases cancer risk. 92

Vegetables decrease cancer risk. 93

Fruits decrease cancer risk 94

Legumes decrease cancer risk 95

Whole grain and fiber decrease cancer risk 96

Vitamin D protects from cancer 97

Key takeaways on cancer. 98

OBESITY & OVERWEIGHT **100**

High BMI cuts life expectancy. 101

Increase in BMI affects health negatively even in the normal range 102

BMI and cholesterol levels are linked. 103

Weight loss diets work ... initially 104

Alternate-day fasting lowers weight 105

Whole foods have high satiety 107

Sleep deprivation causes overeating 108

BMI is consistently normal on plant-based diets 109

Key takeaways on BMI 110

PART II: INTERPRETATION **112**

Targets 115

Means. 119

Fasting. 126

Protein on a plant-based diet. 130

Evidence on saturated fats 131

Comparison to other diets 133

Adapting to your new diet 138

EPILOGUE **143**

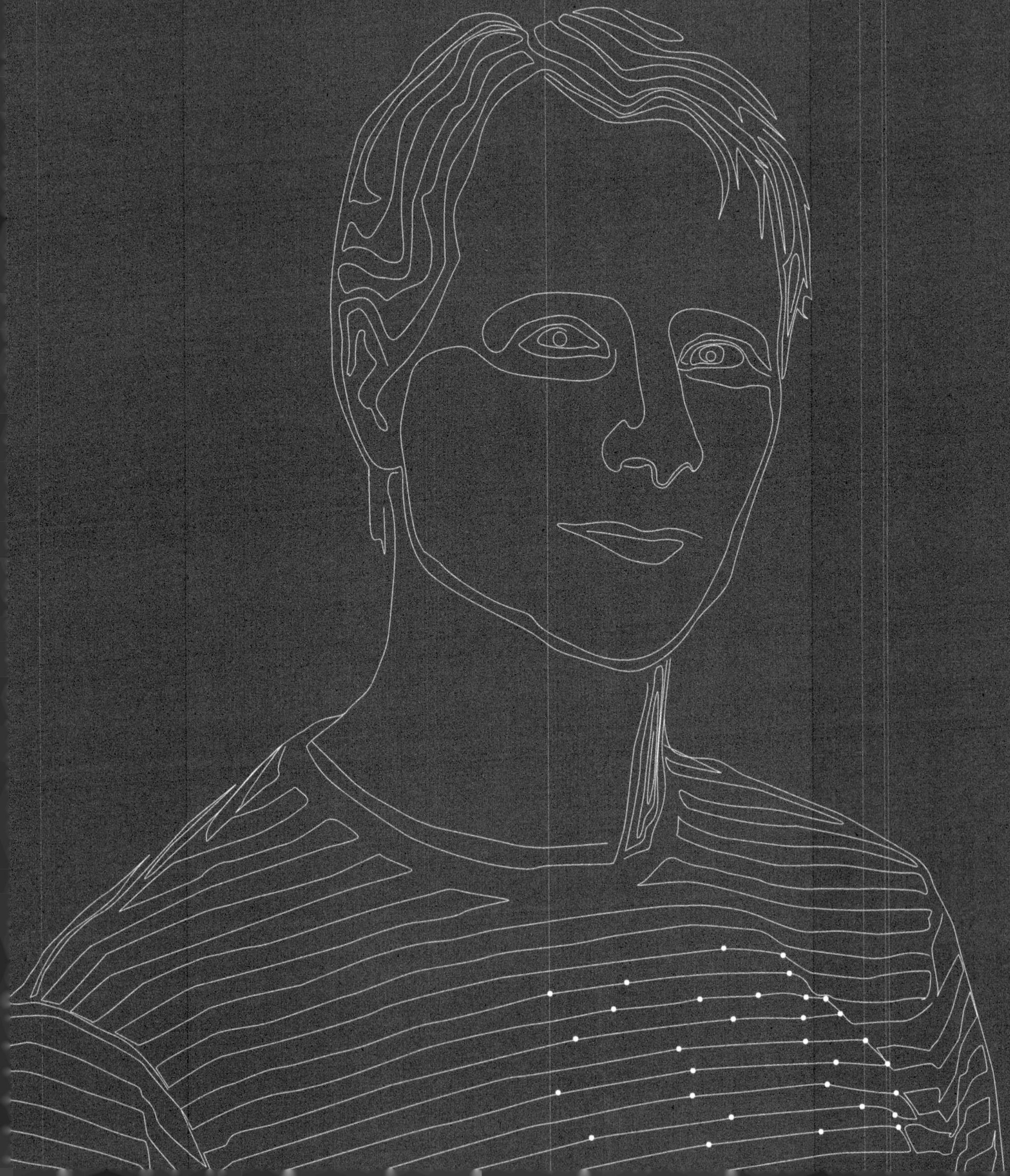

PROLOGUE

This book started as a personal quest to understand how diet affects our health. As a research scientist, I had long been dissatisfied with most diet books that offer ample advice but present little evidence to back their guidance. Which authors can we trust when one book recommends a diet with plenty of whole grains and another book recommends a Paleo diet with no grains? It seems that there are plenty of books promoting every diet ever invented, but it is hard to find a single source of information informed by objective data.

In addition to an academic dissatisfaction with the prevailing offerings, I had a personal urgency to change my diet. As is typical for a Western male, I had cholesterol hovering around 200 mg/dL and my blood pressure had been creeping up over the years. As a young boy, I saw my grandfather suffer from heart disease, which left deep impression on me. I wanted to avoid heart disease and the associated suffering if at all possible. I needed to change my trajectory and I wanted to know if there was an optimal diet that would offer the best chance for a healthy life.

This book is the outcome of reading hundreds of scientific papers. The studies show that it is indeed possible to avoid heart disease by proper diet. And the same diet can also significantly reduce diabetes and cancer risk. Much of the research is new, less than 10 years old and it is not yet incorporated in nutritional guidelines. The data gathered in writing this book has transformed my life. I was able to lower my cholesterol level by 35% from 198 mg/dL to 127 mg/dL, lose 15 lb, and add 3+ years to my life expectancy just by changing my diet. I hope the research data summarized in this book will inspire you to do the same.

Ville Kaajakari, PhD

INTRODUCTION

Diet is a touchy subject. Put strong advocates of a Paleo and vegan diet in a room and you might witness a passionate discussion on dietary philosophy and practice. But one thing is for certain - avoiding the Standard American Diet (SAD) usually means eating healthier. In fact, those not on the SAD have a greater chance of avoiding obesity, type 2 diabetes, heart disease, and cancer.

The Evidence Based Diet covered in this book differs from the other popular diets such as the Paleo diet, vegan diet, or low-carb diet in that it is not based on philosophical arguments on how we should eat. Instead, this work draws from research facts gathered from hundreds of scientific articles. The research evidence shows how to lower body weight, how to avoid common chronic diseases such as heart disease and type 2 diabetes, and how to reduce risk of various types of cancer.

You are probably familiar with the broad outlines of a healthy diet: consume less added sugar and processed food, eat more plant-based food, and reduce consumption of animal protein and fat. And yes, this is what some of the evidence bears out but this book goes further by giving you clear and measurable dietary targets. Whatever your preferred diet is, for example Paleo or vegan, you can use these targets to improve your health. In meeting these targets, you'll stand a good chance at avoiding common chronic diseases such as heart disease and diabetes. And you'll do it confidently, knowing that you're following the latest nutritional research.

Despite knowing what is good for us, we often lack the motivation to stick to eating healthy foods. Rather than repeat the tired advice of "eat your vegetables," this book strives to be inspirational and easy to follow. For example, the most recent research results are summarized in easy to understand figures such as this one[1]:

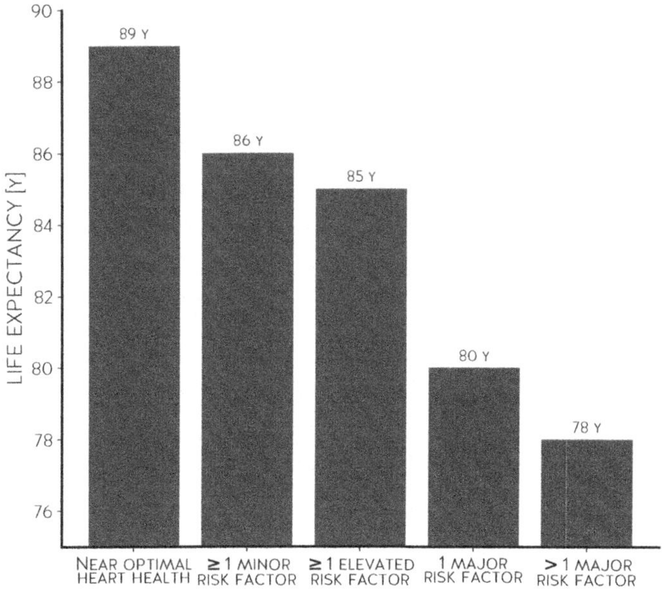

FIG. 1. LIFE EXPECTANCY AND HEART DISEASE RISK FACTORS

Life expectancy with no heart-health risk factors is 89 years but drops to 78 years with more than one major risk factors such as high cholesterol. Lowering cholesterol may be difficult but adding on average 11 years to one's life span can be a major motivator. The research covered in this book will show how diseases such as heart disease and diabetes can largely be avoided by following a healthy diet.

NUTRITIONAL SCIENCE

Nutritional science is one of the hardest research fields as it can be very difficult to prove a causal relationship between the input (diet) and the output (health). There are thousands of different food molecules that affect our health over many decades in complex and nonlinear ways. For example, how can we prove that red meat causes cancer? Ideally, we would have a large pool of identical twins eating two different diets (one with red meat, one without) over their lifetimes and measure the outcome. A study like this is, of course, impossible. Instead, we have data like the following[2]:

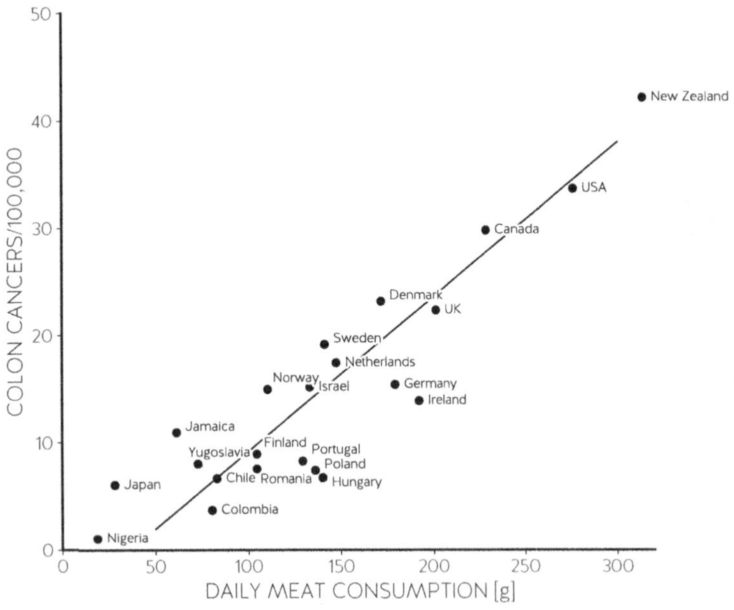

FIG. 2. COLON CANCER RATE AND MEAT CONSUMPTION

It appears that the level of meat intake correlates with the colon cancer incidences in different countries. This correlation, however, is not a proof of causation. It may be possible that some hidden parameter explains the observed correlation. For example, maybe countries with large meat consumption also have large milk consumption. How do we know whether or not meat, milk, or something else entirely is the cause of colon cancer? As we collect more data, the situation becomes clearer. From hundreds of studies analyzing millions of people, it is now established that red meats, and especially processed meats, can cause cancer[13].

In 50-100 years, we will probably know a lot more about nutrition, but we want to know how to stay healthy today.

This gives us some flexibility in adopting research results into the best eating practices. Governmental authorities such as the World Health Organization (WHO) have to balance multiple interests when writing dietary guidelines. This prevents them from issuing advice for example about meat, milk, or tobacco without overwhelming evidence. As private citizens, we do not need to prove everything beyond a reasonable doubt. For example, in population studies, people who regularly eat nuts have less heart disease, but we have limited evidence from clinical trials. The evidence may not be enough for government bodies to include nuts in nutritional guidelines, but it may be enough evidence to make an informed, individual choice to eat nuts.

Similarly, refined carbohydrates are linked to diabetes and cancer. There is not yet sufficient information to make a clear recommendation about the "safe" consumption level for refined carbohydrates, but as individuals, we can choose to eat less of processed foods. In practice, the evidence presented in this book shows that we should eat even more plant-based food than government bodies like the World Health Organization (WHO) currently recommend.

BOOK OUTLINE

The book is organized in two parts.
In Part I we cover scientific evidence on how to:

1} Reduce the risk of heart disease close to zero.

2} Reduce the risk of cancer by more than 30%.

3} Avoid diabetes.

4} Obtain and maintain ideal body mass index (BMI).

Part I consists of research findings that are summarized in easy-to-understand pages such as the following:

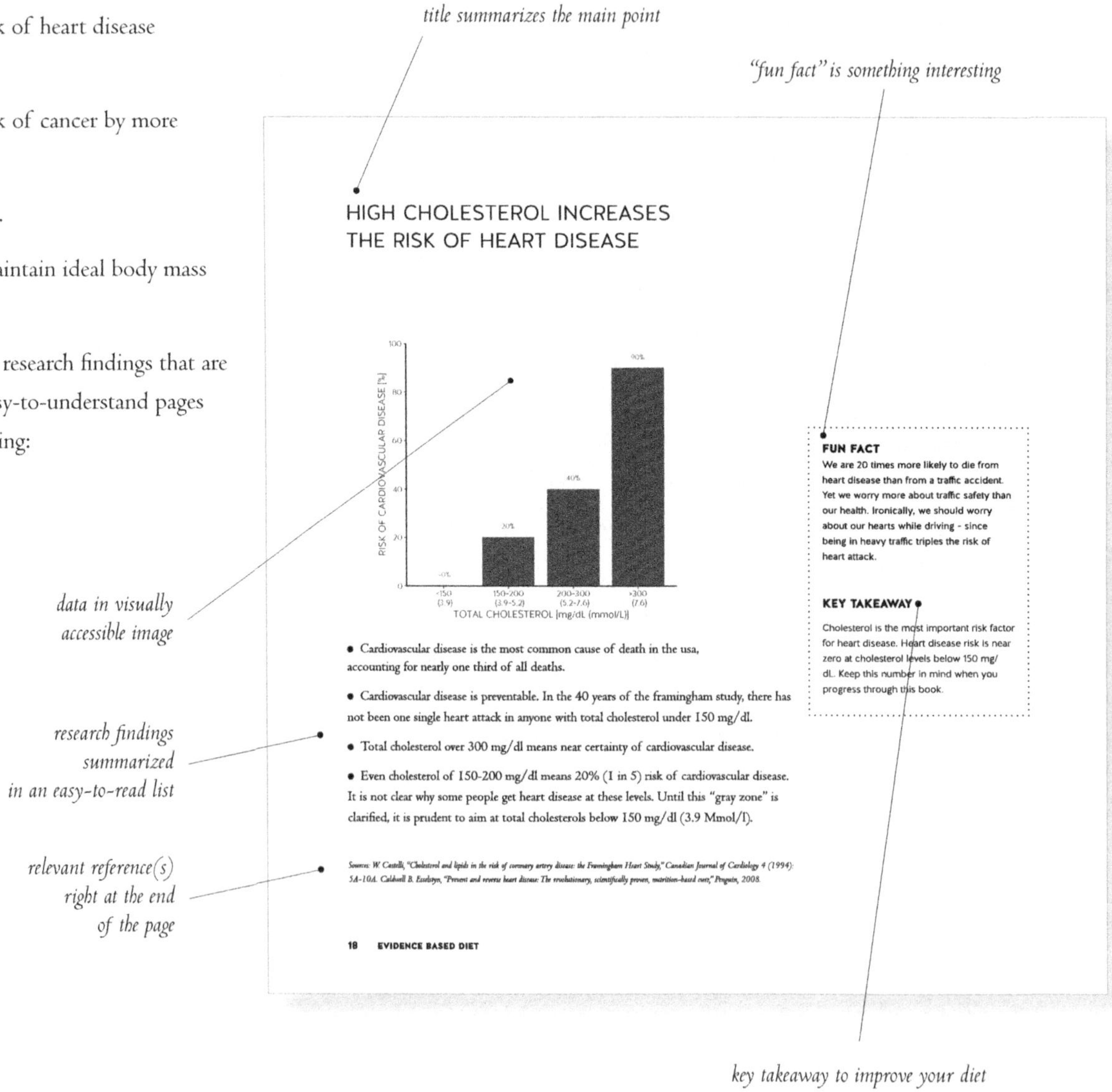

Each page is a self-contained unit that will have a title that summarizes the main point, an informative figure, and summary of the research findings in an easy to read format. The relevant references are given right at the end of the page so there is no need to jump to endnotes if you want search for more details.

In the second part of this book, the evidence presented in Part I is combined to give concise diet guidelines. We will set clear health targets and nutritional means to reach these targets. If you follow this Evidence Based Diet, you will know that you are eating the healthiest diet according to the latest research.

As the research is presented in self-contained units, you can read the book in any order and jump around in the book depending on your priorities. For example, if you are not interested in heart health right now, you can jump directly to the chapter on cancer. Or, if research facts bore you at the moment, you can jump directly to Part II for diet guidelines and then come back to see how the guidelines are supported by the evidence.

DISCLAIMER

In brief: the author is not your doctor and is not offering medical advice.
Full disclaimer below.

This book is not intended as a substitute for the medical advice of physicians. The reader should regularly consult a physician in matters relating to his/her health and particularly with respect to any symptoms that may require diagnosis or medical attention.

Nutrition is ever-evolving science. New research brings about changes in nutrition recommendations. The author is presenting information about nutritional research known at the time of publication. However, in view of the possibility of human error, omission, or changes in medical sciences, neither the author nor the publisher nor any other party who has been involved in the preparation or publication of this work warrants that the information contained herein is in every respect accurate or complete, and they are not responsible for any errors or omissions or for the results obtained from the use of such information.

The Food and Drug Administration has not evaluated any of the statements made in this book. This book is educational and not intended to diagnose, treat, cure, or prevent any disease.

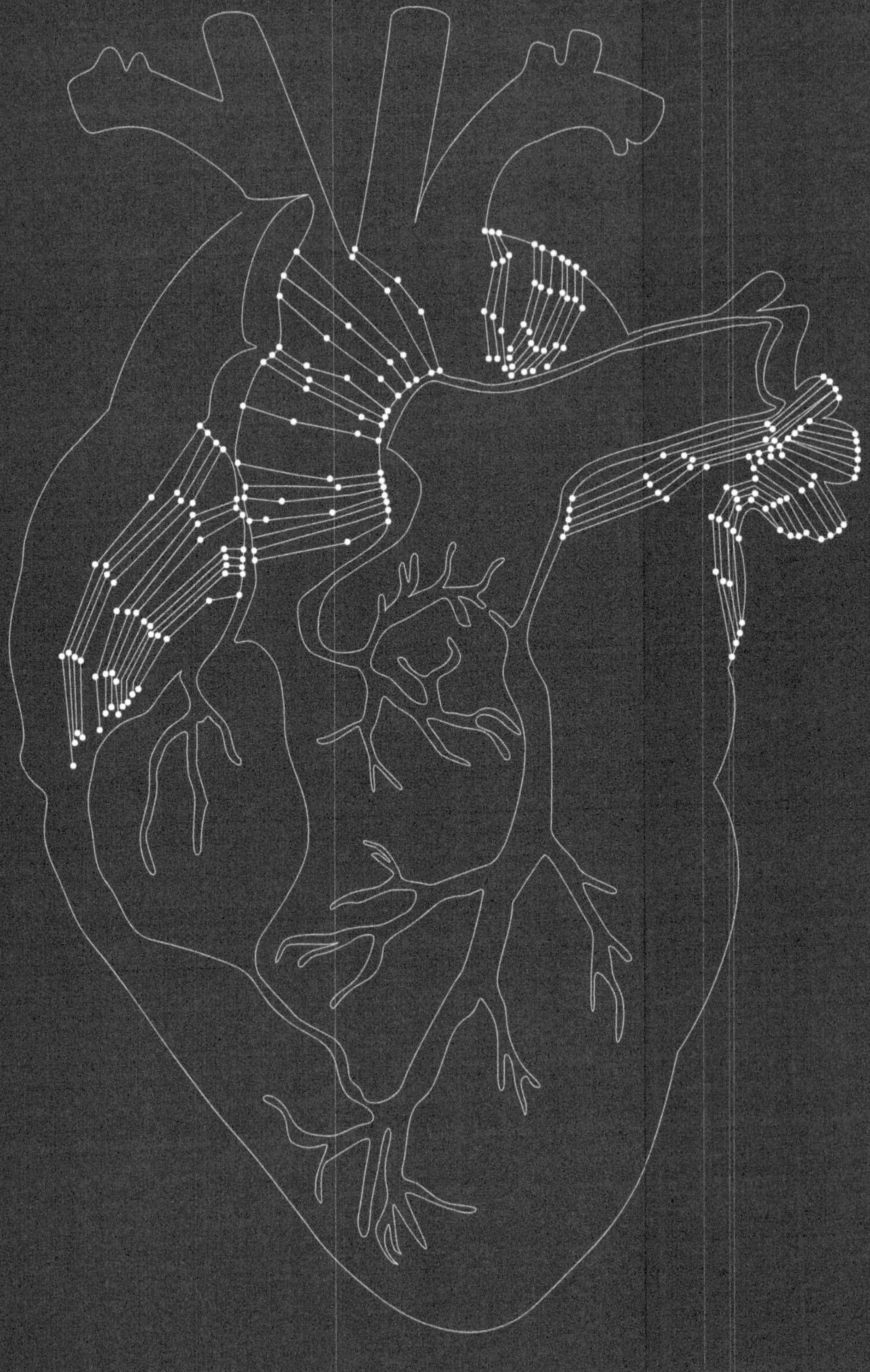

THE EVIDENCE

PART I

The evidence in this book satisfies the following criteria:

- The research outcome must be clear, repeatable, and supported by multiple lines of evidence.
- The results must be significant.

The example of eating nuts satisfies these criteria: First, the evidence is widely supported by population studies and clinical trials. Second, eating nuts has significant positive impact on both cholesterol and the probability of cardiovascular events.

On the other hand, many interesting nutritional findings are not repeatable and/or significant. For example, some studies suggest that eating cinnamon daily can slightly improve fasting glucose and lower cholesterol but the effect is not seen in all studies[15]. Studies like this are purposely left out of this book even though there does not seem to be harm in eating cinnamon and there may be some potential benefits. The problem is that by covering hundreds of potentially healthy foods, we would confuse the bigger picture.

By focusing on the big-impact nutritional items, we can cut through the clutter and focus on what is important: eating mostly plant-based, high-quality proteins, carbohydrates, and fats is the key to a healthy diet. We do not need to chase the latest super foods or supplements but can focus, instead, on the basics of enjoying healthy food from common and readily available grocery store ingredients. It really is that simple.

HEART DISEASE

Heart disease is the deadliest lifestyle disease in the Western world. It is a lifestyle disease because it is not transmitted by a virus or bacteria but caused, to a great extent, by what we eat.

We have known since the 1950s that a simple way to avoid heart disease with near certainty is to eat and exercise like farm workers in Uganda[3]. Ugandans were discovered to be free of heart disease whereas even relatively young Westerners had clogged arteries. Alas, the simple advice to eat like Ugandans is understandably ignored - we like the variety and convenience of the modern foods available to us.

Fortunately, we do not need to become Ugandan farm workers to avoid heart disease. We just need to achieve similar cholesterol levels (total cholesterol below 150 mg/dL or 3.9 mmol/L) to minimize the risk of heart disease. In this chapter, we will cover the evidence for the target cholesterol levels and diet options available to achieve optimal heart health.

HIGH CHOLESTEROL INCREASES THE RISK OF HEART DISEASE

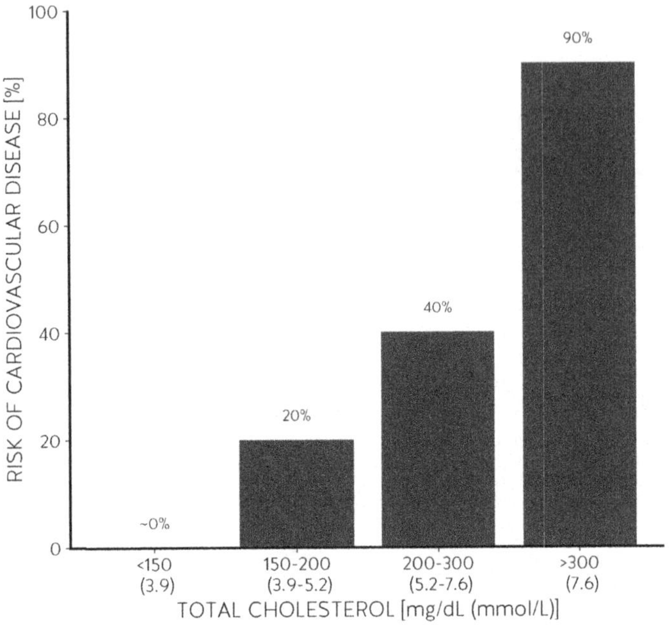

- Cardiovascular disease is the most common cause of death in the USA, accounting for nearly one third of all deaths.
- Cardiovascular disease is preventable. In the 40 years of the Framingham Study, there has not been one single heart attack in anyone with total cholesterol under 150 mg/dl.
- Total cholesterol over 300 mg/dl means near certainty of cardiovascular disease.
- Even cholesterol of 150-200 mg/dl means 20% (1 in 5) risk of cardiovascular disease. It is not clear why some people get heart disease at these levels. Until this "gray zone" is clarified, it is prudent to aim at total cholesterols below 150 mg/dl.

FUN FACT

We are 20 times more likely to die from heart disease than from a traffic accident. Yet we worry more about traffic safety than our health. Ironically, we should worry about our hearts while driving - since being in heavy traffic triples the risk of heart attack.

KEY TAKEAWAY

Cholesterol is the most important risk factor for heart disease. Heart disease risk is near zero at cholesterol levels below 150 mg/dL (3.9 mmol/L). Keep this number in mind when you progress through this book.

W. Castelli, "Cholesterol and lipids in the risk of coronary artery disease: the Framingham Heart Study," Canadian Journal of Cardiology 4 (1994): 5A-10A.

Caldwell B. Esselstyn, "Prevent and reverse heart disease: The revolutionary, scientifically proven, nutrition-based cure," Penguin, 2008.

OPTIMAL LDL CHOLESTEROL IS 50-70 MG/DL

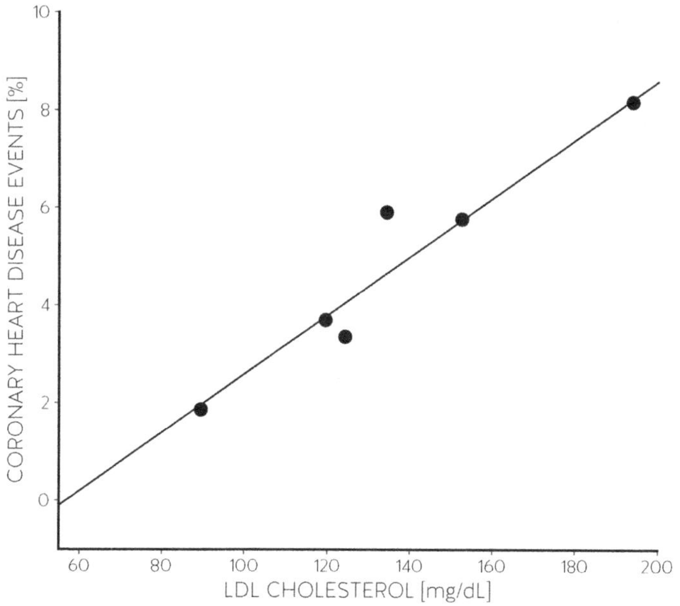

- LDL is labeled as the "bad cholesterol" because high LDL cholesterol increases the risk of cardiovascular disease.
- Multiple lines of evidence demonstrate that the physiologically normal LDL cholesterol level and the threshold for coronary heart disease (CHD) events is approximately 50 to 70 mg/dL (1.3 to 1.7 mmol/L).
- The average LDL level for Americans is approximately 116 mg/dL (3.0 mmol/L).
- LDL level cannot be too low.

O'Keefe, James H., Loren Cordain, William H. Harris, Richard M. Moe, and Robert Vogel, "Optimal low-density lipoprotein is 50 to 70 mg/dL: lower is better and physiologically normal," Journal of the American College of Cardiology 43, No. 11 (2004): 2142-2146.

FUN FACT

The standard treatment guidelines suggest drug therapy to treat cholesterol if one's 10-year risk of developing heart disease is over 20%. The cut-off LDL level for drug therapy is > 130 mg/dL (3.3 mmol/L) if there are no additional risk factors such as diabetes. No treatment is offered to patients with heart disease risk of 10% or less.

FUN FACT

Infants are born with perfect heart health: on average, their total cholesterol is less than 160 mg/dL and LDL is less than 70 mg/dL.

KEY TAKEAWAY

Normal LDL cholesterol is 50-70 mg/dL (1.3-1.7 mmol/L) which is believed to result in a near zero heart disease risk. This is well below the average American LDL cholesterol level of 116 mg/dL (3.0 mmol/L).

APOLIPOPROTEIN MAY BE A SUPERIOR INDICATOR OF CARDIOVASCULAR RISKS COMPARED TO STANDARD CHOLESTEROL MEASUREMENT

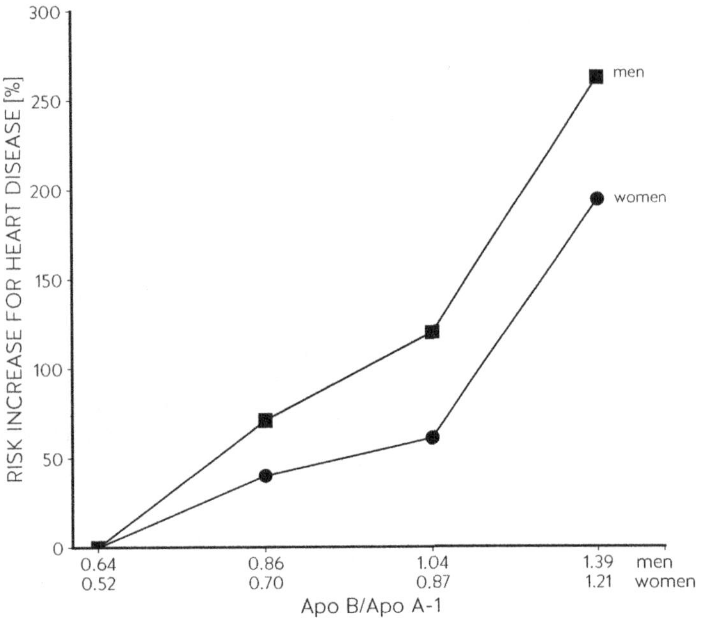

KEY TAKEAWAY

ApoB/apoA-1 ratio is another way to measure lipoprotein levels that also accounts for cholesterol particle size.

- Cholesterol tests measure the lipoprotein densities; however, lipoprotein particle size is also important. A large number of small LDL particles increases heart disease risk more than fewer big particles.
- Apolipoprotein measurement is a newer measurement technique that measures the number of cholesterol particles.
- In large scale studies, apolipoprotein B and apolipoprotein A-I ratio (apoB/apoA-I ratio) is shown to be a better predictor of cardiovascular risks compared to standard cholesterol measurements.

- ApoB/apoA-I ratio of 0.64 (men) and 0.52 (women) indicate the lowest risk of heart disease.

- In direct ultrasonic imaging studies, an apoB/apoA-I ratio >0.74 indicates risk of lipid-related progression of atherosclerosis.

- Although apoB/apoA-I ratio may be a more accurate risk marker than standard cholesterol measurement, it is not yet widely used for screening. Also, whereas we have a wealth of data on the effects of diet on total and LDL cholesterol, we do not yet have much data on the effects of diet and lifestyle on apoB/apoA-I ratio. For now, we will target standard total and LDL cholesterol but we will keep an eye on emerging apoB/apoA-I studies.

G. Walldius, I. Jungner, I. Holme, A. H. Aastveit, W. Kolar, and E. Steiner, "High apolipoprotein B, low apolipoprotein AI, and improvement in the prediction of fatal myocardial infarction (AMORIS study): a prospective study," The Lancet 358, No. 9298 (2001): 2026-2033.

G. Walldius and I. Jungner, "The apoB/apoA ratio: a strong, new risk factor for cardiovascular disease and a target for lipid-lowering therapy - a review of the evidence," Journal of Internal Medicine 259, No. 5 (2006): 493-519.

HEART DISEASE RISK FACTORS DRAMATICALLY AFFECT LIFE EXPECTANCY

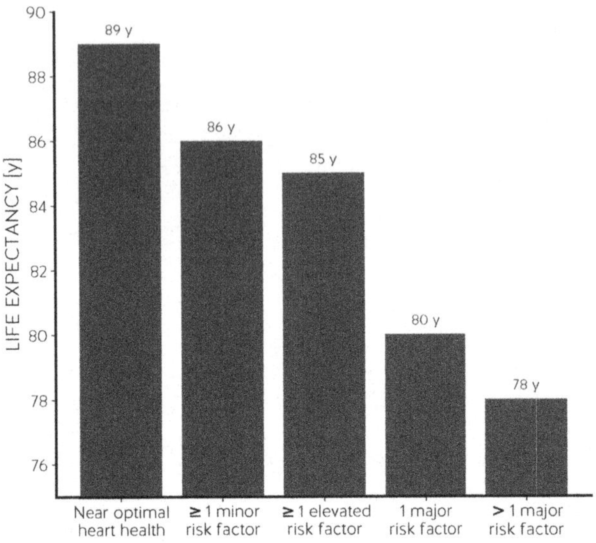

- Median life expectancy for a 50-year old male is heavily dependent on risk factors for cardiovascular disease. Two or more major risk factors lower the median life expectancy by 11 years.

- Near optimal heart health is defined as:

  total cholesterol <180 mg/dL (<4.65 mmol/L)

  blood pressure <120 mmHg (systolic) and <80 mmHg (diastolic)

  nonsmoker

  non-diabetic

FUN FACT

In cultures where heart disease is rare, blood pressure remains normal (below 120 mmHg systolic and 80 mmHg diastolic) throughout one's life.

KEY TAKEAWAY

Heart disease risk factors dramatically affect life expectancy. By controlling these risk factors, average American could increase life expectancy by three years or more.

- Minor risk factors are:

    total cholesterol of 180 to 199 mg/dL (4.65 to 5.15 mmol/L)

    systolic blood pressure of 120 to 139 mmHg, diastolic blood pressure of 80 to 89 mmHg

- Elevated risk factors are:

    total cholesterol 200 to 239 mg/dL (5.16 to 6.19 mmol/L)

    systolic blood pressure of 140 to 159 mm Hg, diastolic blood pressure of 90 to 99 mmHg

- Major risk factors are:

    total cholesterol >240 mg/dL (>6.20 mmol/L)

    systolic blood pressure of >160 mmHg, diastolic blood pressure of > 100 mmHg

    smoker

    diabetic

D. Lloyd-Jones, E. P. Leip, M. G. Larson, R. B. d'Agostino, A. Beiser, P. WF Wilson, P. A. Wolf, and D. Levy, "Prediction of lifetime risk for cardiovascular disease by risk factor burden at 50 years of age," Circulation 113, No. 6 (2006): 791-798.

DIABETES INCREASES CARDIOVASCULAR MORTALITY

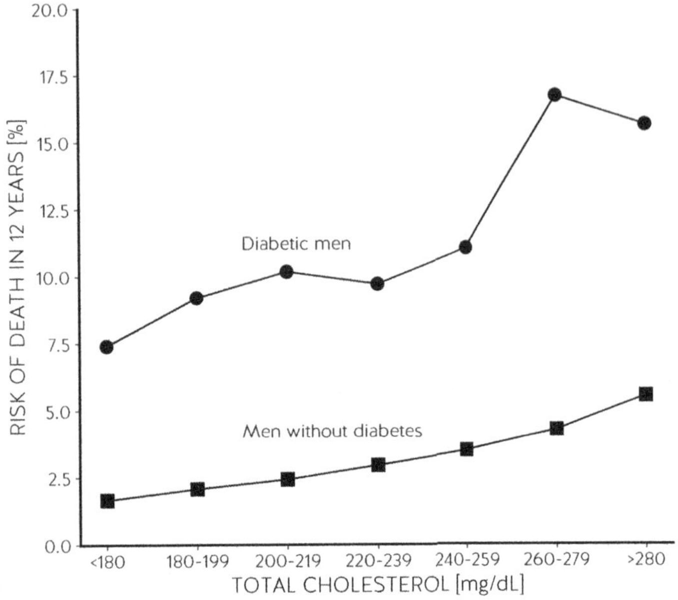

KEY TAKEAWAY
Type-2 diabetes is the biggest risk factor for heart disease.

- Type-2 diabetes dramatically increases heart disease death rates.
- A diabetic, 48-year-old man with the cholesterol level of 200 mg/dL, has 1 in 10 risk of dying by age of 60. For non-diabetic, the death risk is less than 2.5%.
- Avoiding type-2 diabetes is the single most important factor in avoiding death by cardiovascular disease.
- We will cover how to avoid type-2 diabetes separately in the Diabetes chapter.

J. Stamler, O. Vaccaro, J. D. Neaton, and D. Wentworth, "Diabetes, other risk factors, and 12-yr cardiovascular mortality for men screened in the Multiple Risk Factor Intervention Trial," Diabetes Care 16, No. 2 (1993): 434-444.

VEGETARIAN DIET LOWERS CHOLESTEROL

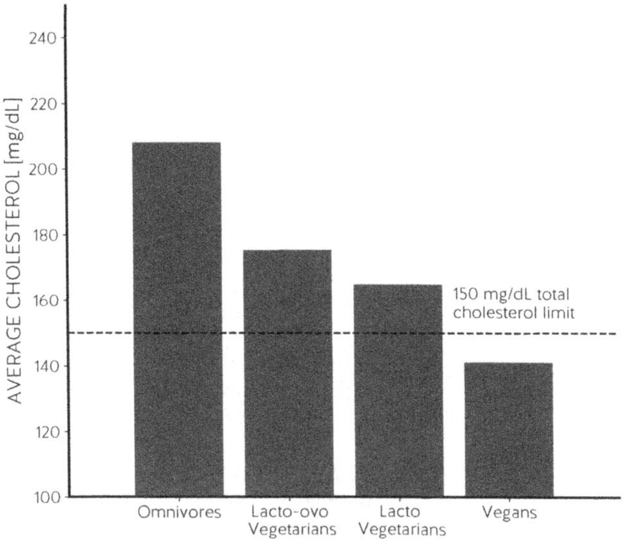

FUN FACT

Vegan is a relatively new term as it was coined in 1994 by Vegan Society founder Donald Watson.

KEY TAKEAWAY

Vegan diet is the only Western diet that consistently achieves a total cholesterol level of less than 150 mg/dL, which minimizes the risk of cardiovascular disease.

- Vegetarian and especially vegan diet achieves low cholesterol levels.

  Vegan diet includes only plants.

  Lacto vegetarian diet also includes dairy products.

  Lacto-ovo vegetarian diet includes dairy and eggs.

- Even in modern society, it is possible to achieve total cholesterol level less than 150 mg/dL that minimizes the risk of cardiovascular disease.
- No difference is reported in the "good cholesterol" (HDL) between the different diet groups.
- There is variation among individuals within each diet and a vegan diet is not a guarantee of optimal cholesterol. This makes sense: a diet consisting of white bread and potato chips is technically "vegan" but it is not healthy.

S. G. De Biase, S. F. Fernandes, R. J. Gianini, and J. L. G. Duarte, "Vegetarian diet and cholesterol and triglycerides levels," Arquivos Brasileiros de Cardiologia 88, No. 1 (2007): 35–39.

AFFLUENT DIET RAISES CHOLESTEROL IN ONE WEEK

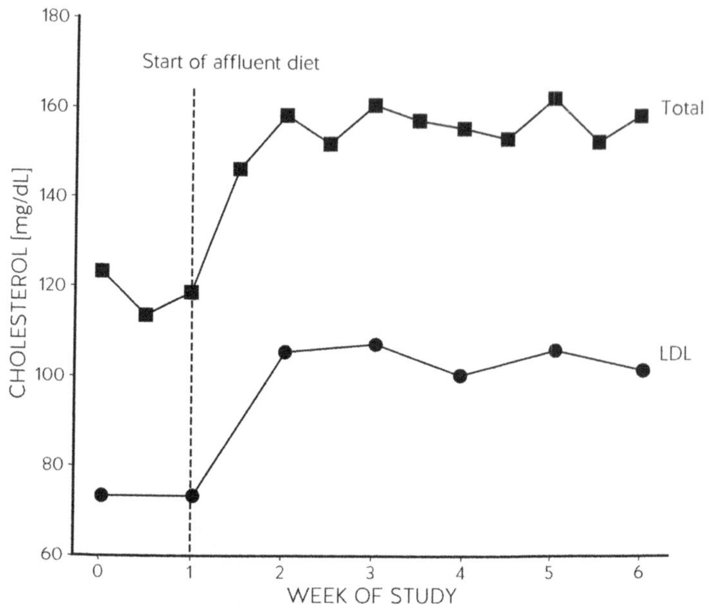

FUN FACT
Many Indigenous Cultures are completely free of heart disease.

KEY TAKEAWAY
The human body responds quickly to diet changes. A typical western diet can raise cholesterol within one week.

- Tarahumara Indians in Mexico who eat traditional diet have excellent cardiovascular health. Their total cholesterol level is less than 130 mg/dL (3.4 mmol/L) and LDL cholesterol is less than 80 mg/dL (2.1 mmol/L).
- The traditional diet for Tarahumara Indians consists of mainly corn and beans, other vegetables and fruits, and small quantities of game, fish, and eggs.
- In a research study, Tarahumara Indians were introduced to a typical, North-American "affluent diet" for 5 weeks. The affluent diet included refined flours, sugar, cheese, butter, eggs, and soft drinks.
- When introduced to the affluent diet, the cholesterol level shot up within one week.

M. P. McMurry, M. T. Cerqueira, S. L. Connor, and W. E. Connor, "Changes in lipid and lipoprotein levels and body weight in Tarahumara Indians after consumption of an affluent diet," New England Journal of Medicine 325, No. 24 (1991): 1704-1708.

CHOLESTEROL LEVEL FOR INDIGENOUS PEOPLE IS BELOW 150 MG/DL

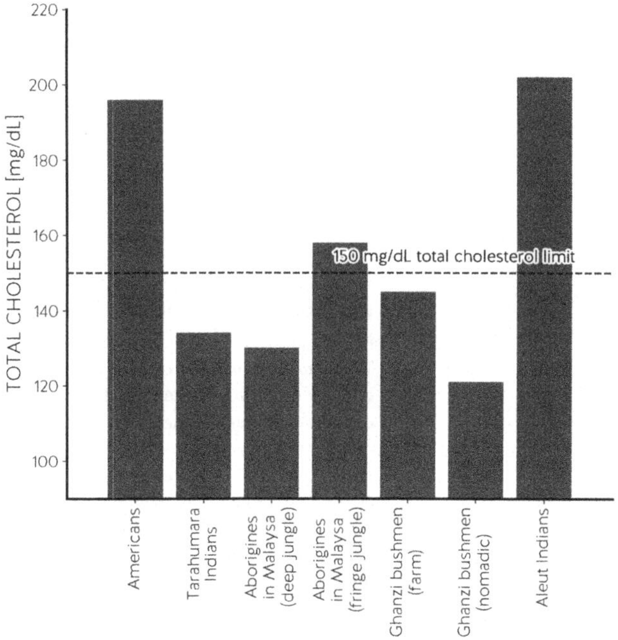

- Cholesterol level for many Indigenous People is below 150 mg/dL (3.9 mmol/L), which is significantly less than the 192 mg/dL (5.0 mmol/L) level of average Americans.
- Cardiovascular disease (CVD) is almost non-existent among Indigenous People with cholesterol levels below 150 mg/dL (3.9 mmol/L) even though they consume some animal products:

> Cerqueira *et al.* write of the Tarahumara Indians of Mexico: "The Tarahumaras are renowned for extraordinary physical fitness and endurance as long-distance runners. Maize was their main staple, meat consumption was rare. Beans of many varieties were a notable part of their diet. "

> Burns-Cox *et al.* write of aborigines in West Malaysia: "The aborigines are thin, extremely fit physically, and for many centuries have lived in the dense hilly jungles

FUN FACT

Contrary to the often heard myth, Inuit are not free of heart disease. This myth was started in 1970s by Danish researchers who noted that Inuit cholesterol levels were about 10% lower than for the average Danes at the time; however, Inuit cholesterol levels hover around 200 mg/dL and Inuits suffer from heart disease. Despite being debunked, the "healthy Inuit myth" is still promoted by the fish oil supplement industry.

KEY TAKEAWAY

Cholesterol levels for Indigenous People that are free of heart disease is below 150 mg/dL. This level also results in near zero heart disease also in Western studies.

of central West Malaysia. Their diet consists chiefly of hand-milled rice as a staple, supplemented with cassava, millet, maize, fish, and fruit, nearly all of which they grow or gather themselves."

Wyndham writes of Ghanzi bushmen: "The Bushmen are still nomadic hunters and live a life which is probably close to that of our Stone Age ancestors. Both the male and the female lead active physical lives. The male tracks the game which he shoots with a bow and poisoned arrows. The female spends her days collecting berries, roots, and water. The staple diet consists of roots, bulbs, and berries. Occasionally there is a kill, and in consequence there is a surfeit of protein in the camp for a few days."

In contrast, Aleut Indians living in the Arctic have cholesterol levels over 200 mg/dL (5.2 mmol/L). Aleut Indians are relatives of Inuit and eat mainly sea foods. Garn and Gertler write: "The Aleut diet is based on fish; the principal year-round staple being salmon, fresh, dried or smoked. Eggs, milk and butter are largely missing from the diet, as are leafy vegetables, except for one summer month."

- Low meat intake may be a contributing factor for the low cholesterol levels among some Indigenous People. Additional factors protecting Indigenous People from heart disease include:

  high levels of mono and poly unsaturated fats

  low Omega-6/Omega-3 fatty acid ratio

  high intakes of antioxidants, fiber, and vitamins

  low salt intake

  daily exercise

  periodic fasting

  no processed food and refined carbohydrates

  no smoking

- When Indigenous People come in contact with the Western diet, their cholesterol levels and heart-disease incidence rate usually increase to Western levels.

FUN FACT
Maasai people in Kenya and Tanzania are often brought up as a counter example of a healthy diet based on animal products. Maasai diet consist largely of milk, blood, and some meat. Despite the diet, Maasai are largely free from heart disease deaths; however, Maasai experience thickening of arteries and coronary artery disease at rates comparable to Americans. It is speculated that their extreme physical fitness and short life span (most Maasai die before age 60 due to illness or violence) play a part in explaining the lack of cardiovascular deaths.

Source: R. B. Wallace, M. D. Malinow, and H. R. Casdorph, "The plasma lipids, lipoproteins, and diet of the Tarahumara Indians of Mexico," The American Journal of Clinical Nutrition 31 (1978): 1131-1142.

M. T. Cerqueira, M. McMurry Fry, and W. E. Connor, "The food and nutrient intakes of the Tarahumara Indians of Mexico," The American Journal of Clinical Nutrition 32, No. 4 (1979): 905-915.

C. J. Burns-Cox, Y. H. Chong, and R. Gillman, "Risk factors and the absence of coronary heart disease in aborigines in West Malaysia," British Heart Journal 34, No. 9 (1972): 953-958.

C. H. Wyndham, "Southern African ethnic adaptation to temperature and exercise," In Baker, Paul T., and Joseph Sidney Weiner (eds), The Biology of Human adaptability, Clarendon (1966): 204.

S. M. Garn and M. M. Gertler, "Serum Cholesterol of Aleut," Canadian Medical Association Journal 64, No. 4 (1951): 338-340.

P. T. Bjerregaard, K. Young, and R. A. Hegele, "Low incidence of cardiovascular disease among the Inuit-what is the evidence?," Atherosclerosis 166, No. 2 (2003): 351-357.

G. V Mann, A. Spoerry, M. Gary, and D. Jarashow, "Atherosclerosis in the Masai," American Journal of Epidemiology 95, No. 1 (1972): 26-37.

HIGH GLYCEMIC INDEX FOODS INCREASE HEART DISEASE RISK

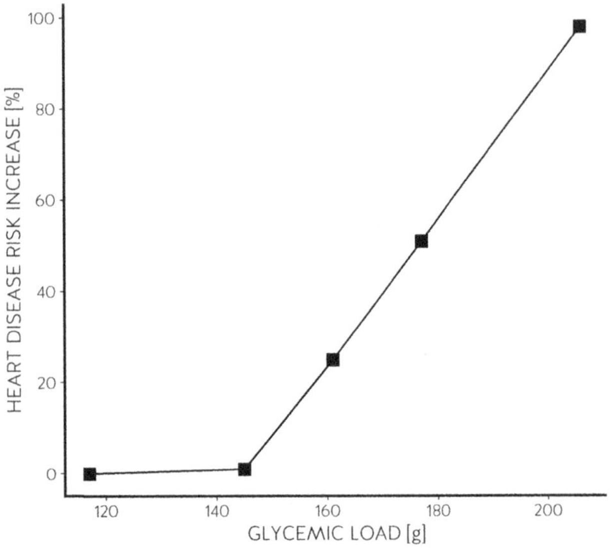

- Glycemic Index (GI) measures how food affects blood sugar levels. A diet with a high glycemic index raises blood sugar levels more than diet with a low glycemic index.
- Glycemic load is the net effect of food's glycemic index and quantity of carbohydrates.
- Risk of heart disease increases with high glycemic load diet.
- High glycemic load diet increases triglyceride and total cholesterol levels.
- High glycemic index foods include glucose (dextrose, grape sugar), high fructose corn syrup, white bread, white rice, corn flakes, extruded breakfast cereals, and white potatoes.

FUN FACT

The Atkins diet, low-carb diet, and whole food plant based diets are variations of a low glycemic index diet.

KEY TAKEAWAY

Avoiding sugar is smart but one should also moderate the intake of highly processed grains such as white rice, bread, and pasta that have high glycemic index and quickly raise blood glucose levels. Eating whole plants is a good way to achieve a low glycemic index diet.

- Low glycemic index foods include beans (black, pinto, kidney, lentil, peanut, chickpea), small seeds (sunflower, flax, pumpkin, poppy, sesame, hemp), walnuts, cashews, most whole intact grains (durum/spelt/kamut wheat, millet, oat, rye, rice, barley), most vegetables, most fruits (peaches, strawberries, mangos), mushrooms, and chilies.

S. Liu, W. C. Willett, M. J. Stampfer, F. B. Hu, M. Franz, L. Sampson, C. H. Hennekens, and J. E. Manson, "A prospective study of dietary glycemic load, carbohydrate intake, and risk of coronary heart disease in US women," The American Journal of Clinical Nutrition 71, No. 6 (2000): 1455-1461.

D. S. Ludwig, "The glycemic index: physiological mechanisms relating to obesity, diabetes, and cardiovascular disease," Journal of American Medical Association 287, No. 18 (2002): 2414-2423.

Y. Amano, K. Kawakubo, J. S. Lee, and A. C. Tang, "Correlation between dietary glycemic index and cardiovascular disease risk factors among Japanese women," European Journal of Clinical Nutrition 58, No. 11 (2004): 1472-1478.

FRUIT AND VEGETABLES PROTECT FROM HEART DISEASE

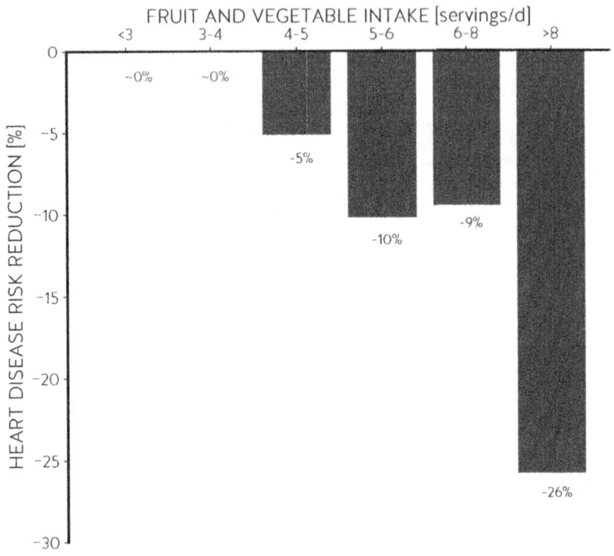

- Fruit and vegetable consumption decreases the risk of coronary heart disease. The more fruit and vegetables one consumes, the lower one's risk of coronary heart disease.
- Vegans and vegetarians also benefit from increasing their fruit and vegetable intake.
- The benefits of increasing fruit and vegetable consumption is not fully explained by the corresponding reduction in meat intake. The results hold even after adjusting for meat intake.
- No single fruit or vegetable is significantly more protective than any other.

FUN FACT

USDA Dietary Guidelines recommend at least 5 servings of fruits and vegetables daily which is not enough to maximize the benefits. Even so, just 30% of Americans meet this low target.

KEY TAKEAWAY

An apple a day does not do much, but more than eight servings of fruits and vegetables per day reduces the risk of heart disease risk by a quarter. The more vegetables you eat, the greater the benefit.

K. J. Joshipura, F. B. Hu, J. E. Manson, M. J. Stampfer,E. B. Rimm, F. E. Speizer, G. Colditz, A. Ascherio, B. Rosner, D. Spiegelman, and W. C. Willett, "The effect of fruit and vegetable intake on risk for coronary heart disease," Annals of Internal Medicine 134, No. 12 (2001): 1106-1114.

P. van't Veer, M. C. Jansen, M. Klerk, and F. J. Kok, "Fruits and vegetables in the prevention of cancer and cardiovascular disease," Public Health Nutrition 3, No. 1 (2000): 103-107.

OAT BRAN LOWER CHOLESTEROL

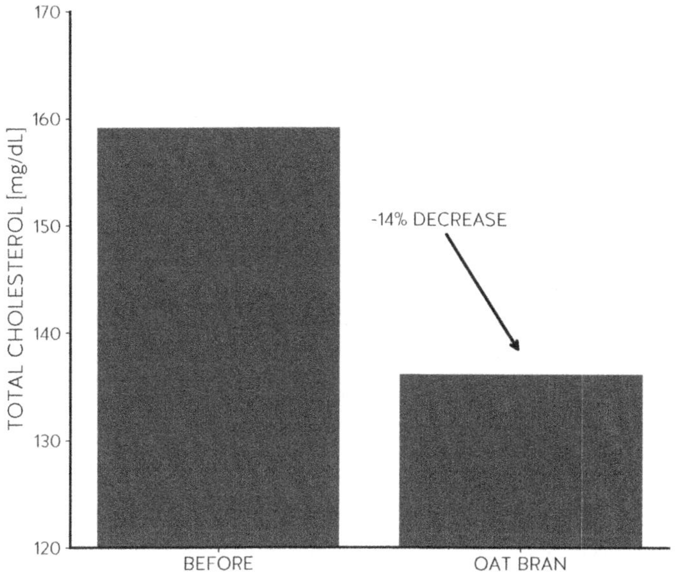

- Oat bran lowers total cholesterol and LDL cholesterol.
- Diet with a daily oat bran intake of 3.5 oz (100 g) lowers total cholesterol by -14% in healthy adults. Similar reduction is also observed in people with high cholesterol levels.

M. Kristensen and S. Bugel, "A diet rich in oat bran improves blood lipids and hemostatic factors, and reduces apparent energy digestibility in young healthy volunteers," European Journal of Clinical Nutrition 65, No. 9 (2011): 1053-1058

R. W. Kirby, J. W. Anderson, B. Sieling, E. D. Rees, W. J. Chen, R. E. Miller, and R. M. Kay, "Oat-bran intake selectively lowers serum low-density lipoprotein cholesterol concentrations of hypercholesterolemic men," The American Journal of Clinical Nutrition 34, No. 5 (1981): 824-829.

FUN FACT

The cholesterol lowering effect of oat bran is partially due to b-glucan. The US Food and Drug Administration allows a claim that oat-containing food products that deliver 3 grams of b-glucan daily can reduce the risk of heart disease. However, b-glucan supplements do not yield the same effect as whole oats. It is usually better to eat whole foods than supplements.

KEY TAKEAWAY

Adding 3.5 oz (about 1 cup) of oats to one's daily diet may significantly lower one's cholesterol level.

WHOLE GRAIN DECREASE HEART DISEASE RISK

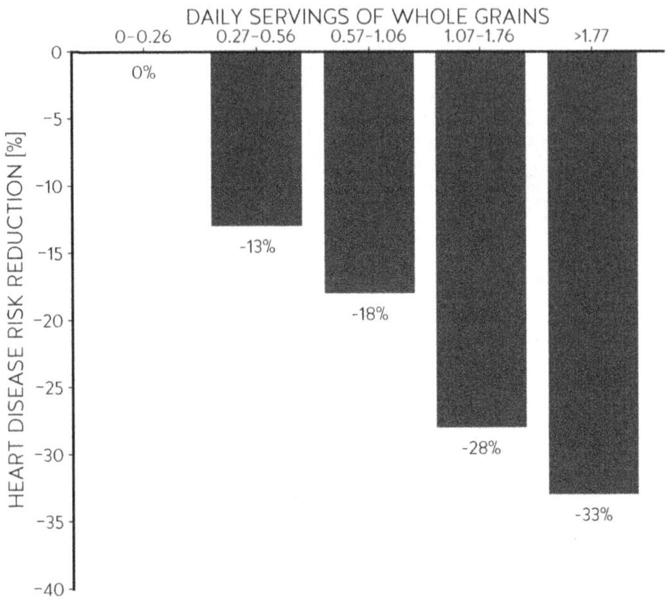

KEY TAKEAWAY
Whole grains, for example whole grain bread, oatmeal, brown rice, and porridge, reduce the risk of heart disease.

- Whole grains reduce the risk of heart disease.
- In contrast, refined grains, such as white flour and white rice, increase the risk of heart disease.
- Whole grains contain dietary fiber, vitamin E, and folate which are associated with reduced risk of heart disease.

S. Liu, M. J. Stampfer, F. B. Hu, E. Giovannucci, E. Rimm, J.A. E. Manson, C. H. Hennekens, and W. C. Willett, "Whole-grain consumption and risk of coronary heart disease: results from the Nurses' Health Study," The American Journal of Clinical Nutrition 70, No. 3 (1999): 412-419.

TRANS FATS INCREASE HEART DISEASE RISK

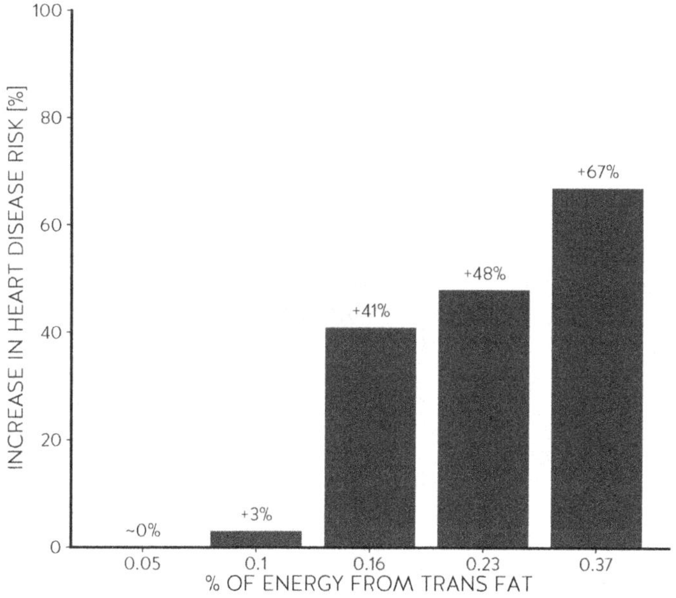

FUN FACT

The average American cholesterol level decreased from an average of 204 mg/dL in 1999-2000 to an average of 192 mg/dL in 2011-2014. This drop is attributed to a reduction of added trans fats in foods.

KEY TAKEAWAY

Trans fats are extremely harmful even in small quantities. Added trans fats are now banned by FDA but trans fats naturally occur in some animal products. Check product labels and avoid products with any trans fats.

- Trans fats are the worst kind of fat. Diets with just 0.2% of energy coming from trans fats increase the risk of heart disease by nearly 50%. In a normal 2,000-calorie diet, 0.2% translates to 0.4 g of trans fat.

- Added trans fats, including partially hydrogenated vegetable oils, are so dangerous that they have been banned in the US by the Food and Drug Administration (FDA) since 2018.

- Even after the ban, some animal products including dairy and meat still naturally contain trans fats. For example, a pepperoni pizza has 2.5 g of trans fat from meat and cheese.

M. Guasch-Ferré et al., "Dietary fat intake and risk of cardiovascular disease and all-cause mortality in a population at high risk of cardiovascular disease," The American Journal of Clinical Nutrition 102, No. 6 (2015): 1563-1573.

TRANS FATS OCCUR NATURALLY IN ANIMAL PRODUCTS

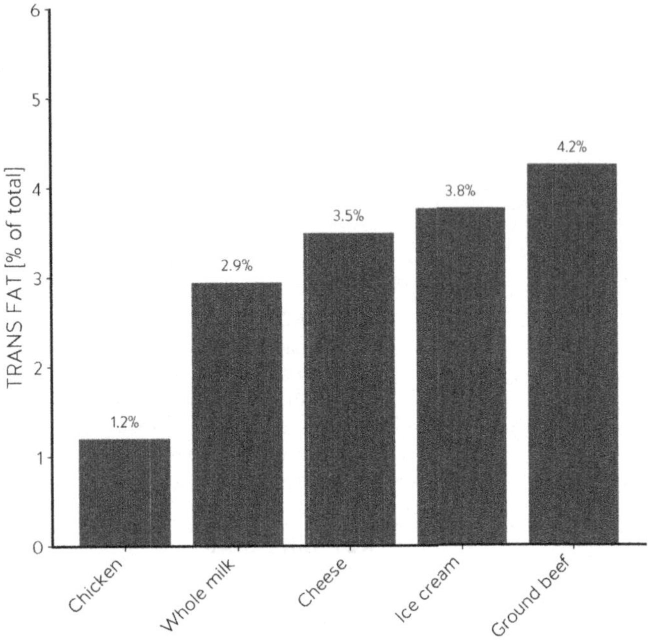

- Trans fats raise your LDL ("bad") cholesterol and lowers your HDL ("good") cholesterol. It is considered the worst kind of fat.
- Health authorities worldwide recommend that consumption of trans fat be reduced to trace amounts.
- Trans fat occurs naturally in many animal products. Meat and dairy products are now the main sources of trans fats.

FUN FACT

A slice of cheese contains 0.3 g of trans fats which is often rounded down to 0 g on the nutritional facts label. This may make some consumers unaware that cheese has trans fats. Just two slices of cheese daily has enough trans fat to increase the risk of heart disease by more than 50%.

KEY TAKEAWAY

Be mindful about foods that naturally contain trans fats. For example, cheese, meats, and ice cream contain trans fat.

FDA Cuts Trans Fat in Processed Foods, Food and Drug Administration, Online: https://www.fda.gov/ForConsumers/ConsumerUpdates/ucm372915.htm

Jacob Exler, Linda Lemar, and Julie Smith, "Fat and Fatty Acid Content of Selected Foods Containing Trans-Fatty Acids," USDA.

MILK FAT INCREASES HEART DISEASE MORTALITY

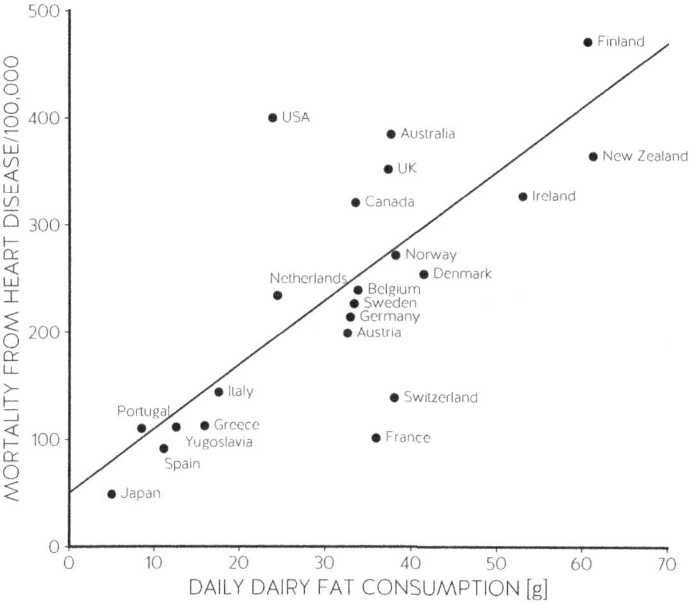

FUN FACT

Butter has about 50% saturated fat and 4% trans fat .

KEY TAKEAWAY

Limit the milk and especially milk fat consumption to minimize the heart disease death risk.

- There is a close correlation between the consumption of dairy fats and the mortality from heart disease among different countries.
- In a landmark trial, carried out in a controlled environment (a hospital in Finland) over a period of 12 years, milk fat was replaced with vegetable oils. This simple change resulted in over 50% reduction in heart disease mortality.

O. Turpeinen, "Effect of cholesterol-lowering diet on mortality from coronary heart disease and other causes," Circulation 59, No. 1 (1979): 1-7.

M. Miettinen, M. Karvonen, O. Turpeinen, R. Elosuo, and E. Paavilainen, "Effect of cholesterol-lowering diet on mortality from coronary heart-disease and other causes: a twelve-year clinical trial in men and women," The Lancet 300, No. 7782 (1972): 835-838.

SATURATED FAT INCREASES CHOLESTEROL LEVELS

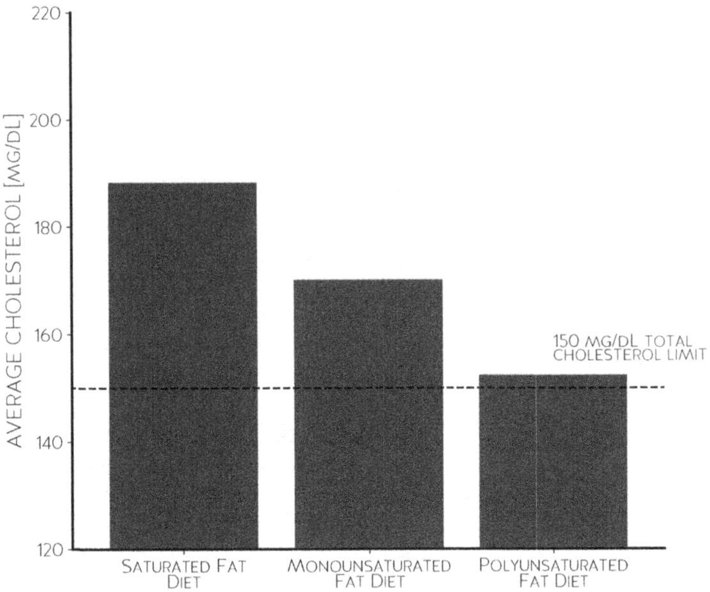

- Saturated fat increases cholesterol levels. Both total and LDL cholesterol levels are increased with a diet high in saturated fats.
- Replacing saturated fats with unsaturated fats, fruits, or vegetables can improve cholesterol levels.
- Replacing saturated fats with refined carbohydrates, however, is not a good idea as refined carbohydrates can raise triglyceride levels and lower the "good" HDL cholesterol.

L. Hodson, C. M. Skeaff, and W. A. Chisholm, "The effect of replacing dietary saturated fat with polyunsaturated or monounsaturated fat on plasma lipids in free-living young adults," European Journal of Clinical Nutrition 55, No. 10 (2001): 908-915.

FUN FACT

Most saturated fats are from animal products but some vegetable oils also contain large quantities of saturated fat. For example, coconut oil is 90% saturated fats.

KEY TAKEAWAY

It is good idea to prefer unsaturated fats (olive oil, avocado oil, or nut oil) over saturated fats (coconut oil, palm oil, butter, and other animal fats).

REPLACING SATURATED FAT UNSATURATED FAT DECREASES HEART DISEASE RISK

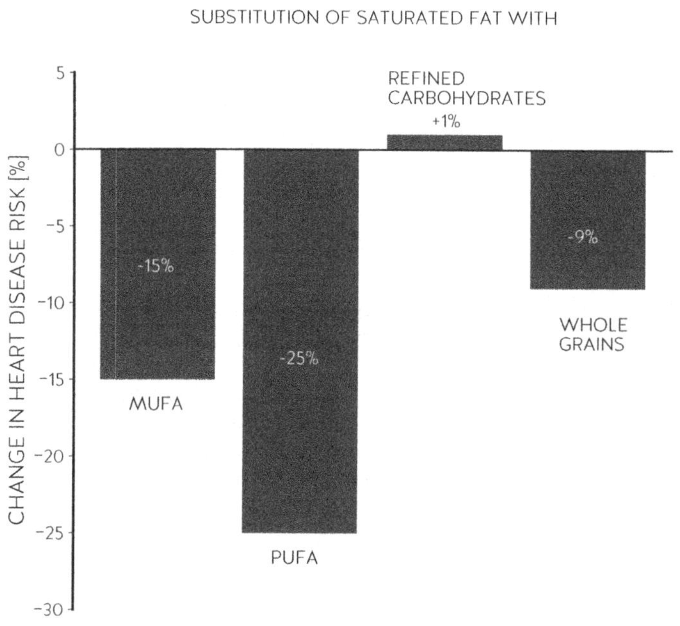

- Saturated fatty acids or saturated fats increase cholesterol levels. Diets high in saturated fat are associated with higher risk of heart disease.
- Reducing saturated fat intake is beneficial if saturated fats are replaced with monounsaturated fatty acids (MUFA), polyunsaturated fatty acids (PUFA), or unprocessed carbohydrates such as fruits, vegetables, and whole grains.
- Replacing saturated fat with refined grains and sugars offers no benefit and may even increase the risk of heart disease.

Y. Li, A. Hruby, A. M. Bernstein, S. H. Ley, D. D. Wang, S. E. Chiuve, L. Sampson, K. M. Rexrode, E. B. Rimm, W. C. Willett, and F. B. Hu, "Saturated fats compared with unsaturated fats and sources of carbohydrates in relation to risk of coronary heart disease: a prospective cohort study," Journal of the American College of Cardiology 66, No. 14 (2015): 1538-1548.

FUN FACT

Global low-fat food market size is over $50B but processed, low-fat foods may not actually be healthy for the heart if they are high in refined carbohydrates such as sugar and starch.

KEY TAKEAWAY

The often repeated advice to avoid saturated fats is valid but saturated fats should be replaced with something healthy. Replacing bacon with a donut may not bring benefits.

UNSATURATED FATS DECREASE THE RISK OF HEART DISEASE

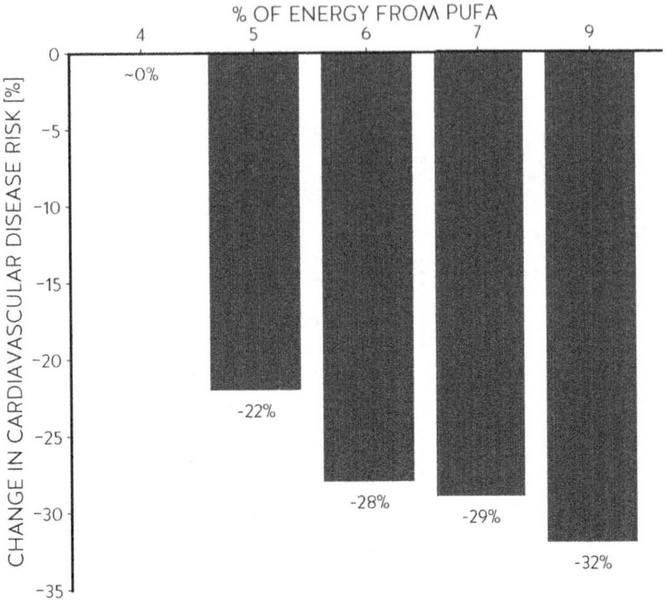

- Not all fats are bad. Mono-unsaturated fatty acids (MUFAs) and polyunsaturated fatty acids (PUFAs) decrease heart disease and mortality risk.
- Some unsaturated fats including Omega-3 and Omega-6 are essential. Humans need, but cannot produce, them.

FUN FACT

We have known since the 1950s that a diet high in unsaturated fats is more effective in lowering cholesterol than a low-fat diet. This fact was forgotten during the low-fat diet craze when all fats, good and bad, were shunned.

KEY TAKEAWAY

It is not necessary to avoid all fats. Diet should be low in trans fats and saturated fats but may contain unsaturated fats. It is still a good idea to moderate all fat use as fat is very energy dense but one does not need to feel guilty of sprinkling some olive oil on salads.

M. Guasch-Ferri, N. Babio, M. A. Martinez-Gonzalez, D. Corella, E. Ros, S. Martin-Peliez, R. Estruch, F. Aris, E. Gimez-Gracia, M. Fiol, J. M. Santos-Lozano, L. Serra-Majem, M. Bulli, E. Toledo, R. Barragin, M. Fiti, A. Gea, and J. Salas-Salvadi, "Dietary fat intake and risk of cardiovascular disease and all-cause mortality in a population at high risk of cardiovascular disease," The American Journal of Clinical Nutrition 102, No. 6 (2015): 1563-1573.

J. M. R. Beveridge, F. Connell, and G. A. Mayer, "Dietary factors affecting the level of plasma cholesterol in humans: the role of fat," Canadian Journal of Biochemistry and Physiology 34, No. 3 (1956): 441-455.

OMEGA-6/OMEGA-3 RATIO MAY BE IMPORTANT FOR HEART HEALTH

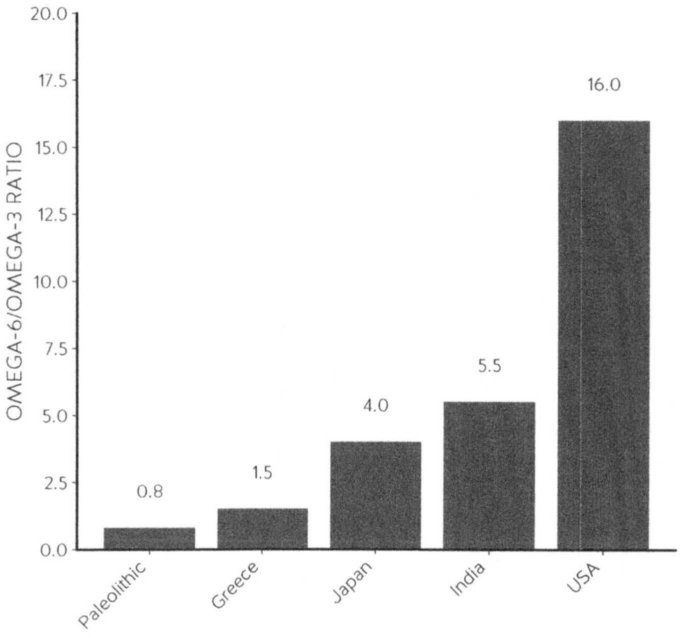

- Omega-3 and Omega-6 are essential fats. Humans need but cannot produce them. A healthy diet should provide both Omega-3 and Omega-6 fats in the right proportion.
- The Western diet has too much Omega-6 in comparison to diets that are associated with a healthy heart.
- The Lyon Heart Study showed that the diet of Crete decreases cardiovascular disease mortality by 70%. An essential part of the study was an increase in Omega-3 and a decrease in Omega-6 to improve the Omega-6/Omega-3 ratio.
- Optimal ratio for Omega-6/Omega-3 intake is between one and three. In the Western diet, the ratio is 16.
- Most industrial vegetable oils such as cottonseed and corn oil are high in Omega-6 but low in Omega-3. Avoid these industrially processed oils.

FUN FACT

Chia seeds or flax seeds, fish, and walnuts are good sources of Omega-3s.

KEY TAKEAWAY

Human needs both Omega-3 and Omega-6 oils in right proportion. Avoid processed vegetable oils that are low in Omega-3s. Olive oil is a good choice as it contains both Omega-3 and Omega-6 oils. In addition, it is a good idea to supplement your diet for example with flaxseed, fish, or walnuts that are high in Omega-3s.

- Olive oil has a better Omega-6/Omega-3 ratio of 9.
- Low to moderate intake of fish – about 1 fish meal per week – is associated with a 50% lower risk sudden death compared to diets with very low fish consumption. This risk reduction is attributed to long chain Omega-3 fatty acids in fish.
- To further increase Omega-3 intake, supplement your diet for example with chia or flax seeds. Flax seed has 3 times more Omega-3 than Omega-6.

A. P. Simopoulos, "Omega-6/Omega-3 essential fatty acid ratio and chronic diseases," Food Reviews International 20, No. 1 (2004): 77-90.

M. de Lorgeril and P. Salen, "Modified Cretan Mediterranean diet in the prevention of coronary heart disease and cancer: an update," World Review of Nutrition and Dietetics 97 (2007): 1-32.

R. Marchioli, F. Barzi, E. Bomba, C. Chieffo, D. Di Gregorio, R. Di Mascio, M. G. Franzosi, E. Geraci, G. Levantesi, A.P. Maggioni, and L. Mantini, "Early protection against sudden death by n-3 polyunsaturated fatty acids after myocardial infarction," Circulation 105, No. 16 (2002): 1897-1903.

Albert, Christine M., Charles H. Hennekens, Christopher J. O'Donnell, Umed A. Ajani, Vincent J. Carey, Walter C. Willett, Jeremy N. Ruskin, and JoAnn E. Manson. "Fish consumption and risk of sudden cardiac death." JAMA 279, no. 1 (1998): 23-28.

FUN FACT

Human cannot convert Omega-6 to Omega-3 or vice versa. Hence, our body cell membranes reflect Omega-6/Omega-3 ratio of our diet. You are what you eat - literally.

HOMOCYSTEINE IS TOXIC TO HEART

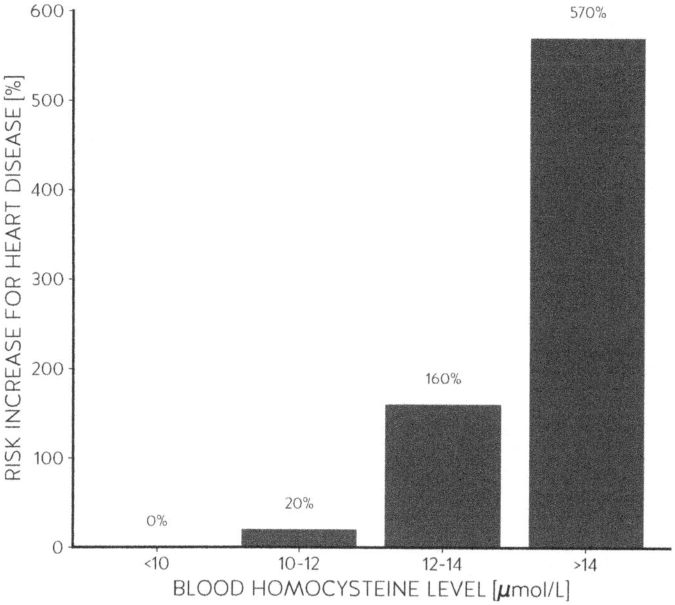

FUN FACT

Low B12 levels and high homocysteine levels may explain why vegans can have fatal heart events even though their cholesterol levels are generally low.

FUN FACT

Folates are found in plant products, especially in green leafy vegetables.

KEY TAKEAWAY

Everyone needs vitamin B12 to dispose toxic homocysteine. Most people do not get enough B12 through their diet. B12 supplementation is a smart idea.

- Homocysteine level is an independent risk factor for heart disease. Homocysteine levels greater than 14 μmol/L increase heart disease risk by six times compared to optimal homocysteine level <10 μmol/L.
- Human body needs both folates and B12 vitamin to remove homocysteine. B12 is produced by bacteria and is also found in animal products.
- Vegans should eat B12 supplements or B12 fortified foods to control homocysteine levels. Some vegans opt for B12 injections.
- Even meat eaters can benefit from B12 supplements and/or B12 fortified foods since the modern diets do not provide optimal B12 intake.

N. Pancharuniti et al., "Plasma homocyst(e)ine, folate, and vitamin B-12 concentrations and risk for early-onset coronary artery disease, The American Journal of Clinical Nutrition" 59, No. 4 (1994): 940-948.

OPTIMAL B12 LEVEL IS ACHIEVED WITH FORTIFIED FOODS OR SUPPLEMENTS

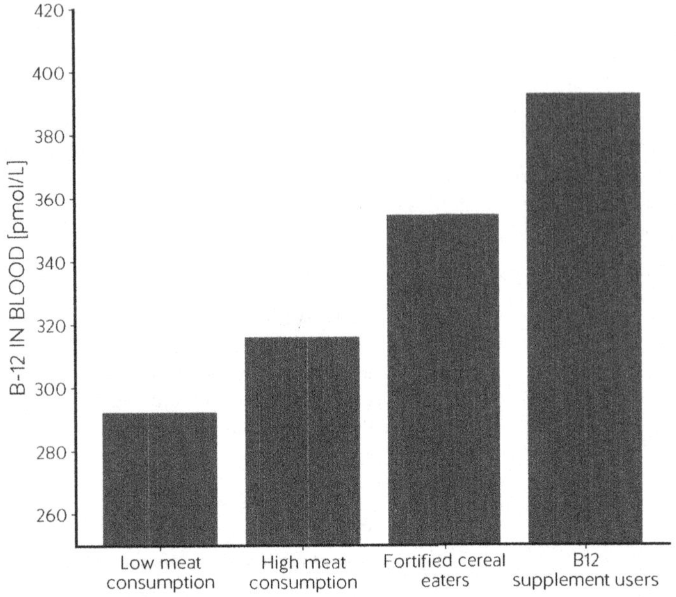

FUN FACT

In factory farming, cows do not obtain sufficient B12 naturally and are given B12 supplements. The "naturally occuring" B12 in meat is no different than the B12 supplements at pharmacy.

KEY TAKEAWAY

In modern diet, optimal B12 levels are achieved only by supplementation. The saturation level is reached with the daily B12 intake of 4-7 μg/day.

- Vitamin B12 is produced by bacteria. It is found in animal products such as meat. Persons eating large amounts of meat have more B12 vitamin in their blood than persons eating only small amount of meat.
- Highest B12 levels are obtained with B12 supplements and fortified foods.
- The daily B12 intake should be 4-7 μg/day to maintain optimal homocysteine level of <10 μmol/L. In modern diets, this level is usually achieved only by supplementation. B12 is water soluble vitamin and higher doses of B12 do not offer additional benefit as they are simply excreted in urine.
- Large meat intake has an adverse effect on cholesterol levels. It is therefore better to obtain B12 from fortified foods or supplements.

- Vegans who do not consume fortified foods or take B12 supplements can suffer from dangerously low B12 levels. This increases fatal heart disease risk and can lead to nerve problems like numbness or tingling, muscle weakness, memory loss, vision loss, and mental problems like depression.

M. V. Bor, K. M. von Castel-Roberts, G. P. Kauwell, S. P. Stabler, R. H. Allen, D. R. Maneval, L: B. Bailey, and E. Nexo, "Daily intake of 4 to 7 ug dietary vitamin B-12 is associated with steady concentrations of vitamin B-12 related biomarkers in a healthy young population," The American Journal of Clinical Nutrition 91, No. 3 (2010): 571-577.

K. Kucker, S. Rich, I. Rosenberg, P. Jacques, G. Dallal, P. W. Wilson, and J. Selbub, "Plasma vitamin B-12 concentrations relate to intake source in the Framingham Offspring study," The American Journal of Clinical Nutrition 71, No. 2 (2000): 514-522.

NUTS LOWER CHOLESTEROL

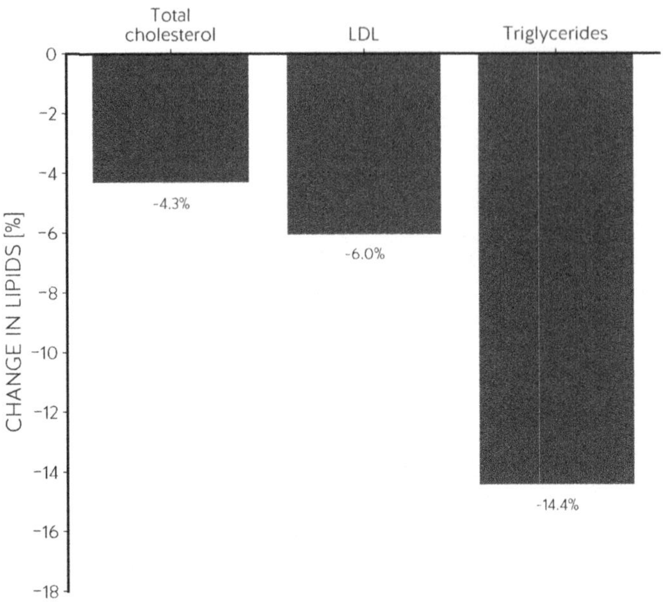

FUN FACT

Pistachios are actually not nuts but fruits. They get their green color from chlorophyll - the same pigment that makes kale green.

KEY TAKEAWAY

Nuts lower cholesterol. It is not nuts to eat them daily.

- Nuts improve blood cholesterol levels.
- Total cholesterol, LDL, and triglycerides are all improved after eating 2.3 oz (66 g) of almonds daily for six weeks. HDL cholesterol is also slightly improved.
- Improvement may be due to monounsaturated fats in nuts. Consuming nut oils offer similar benefits.

D. A. Hyson, B. O. Schneeman, and P. A. Davis, "Almonds and almond oil have similar effects on plasma lipids and LDL oxidation in healthy men and women," The Journal of Nutrition 132, No. 4 (2002): 703-707.

NUTS CAN CUT HEART DISEASE RISK IN HALF

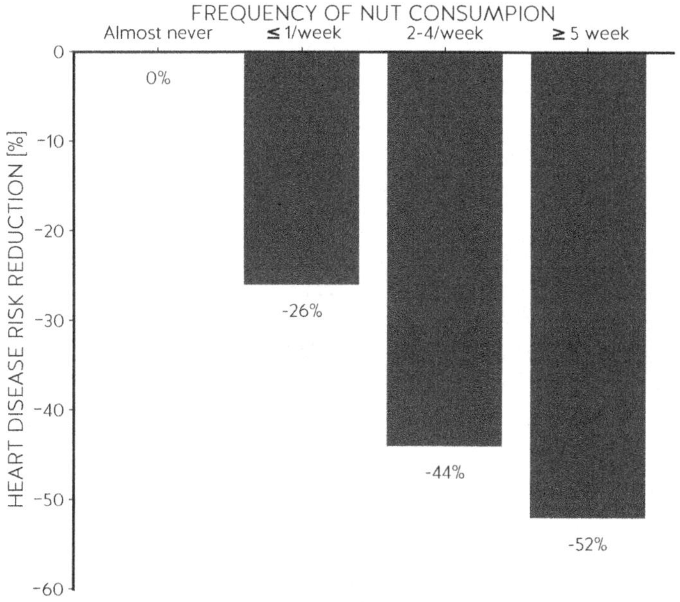

FUN FACT

Peanuts are not true nuts but legumes. But in this study, they count as nuts.

KEY TAKEAWAY

Nuts decrease the risk of heart disease risk. Eat some daily.

- Frequent nut consumption is associated with a significantly reduced risk of coronary heart disease.
- Women who consume nuts >5 times per week have about a 50% lower risk of coronary heart disease than those women who rarely ate nuts. After adjusting for other risk factors such as smoking, nut consumption can decrease coronary heart disease by 35%.
- Population studies show correlation but are not a proof of causation; however, there is little harm and a big potential upside in eating nuts.

F. B. Hu, M. J. Stampfer, J. E. Manson, E. B. Rimm, G. A. Colditz, B. A. Rosner, F. E. Speizer, C. H. Hennekens, and W. C. Willett, "Frequent nut consumption and risk of coronary heart disease in women: prospective cohort study," BMJ: British Medical Journal 317, No. 7169 (1998): 1341-1345.

RED MEAT INCREASES RISK OF DEATH FROM HEART DISEASE

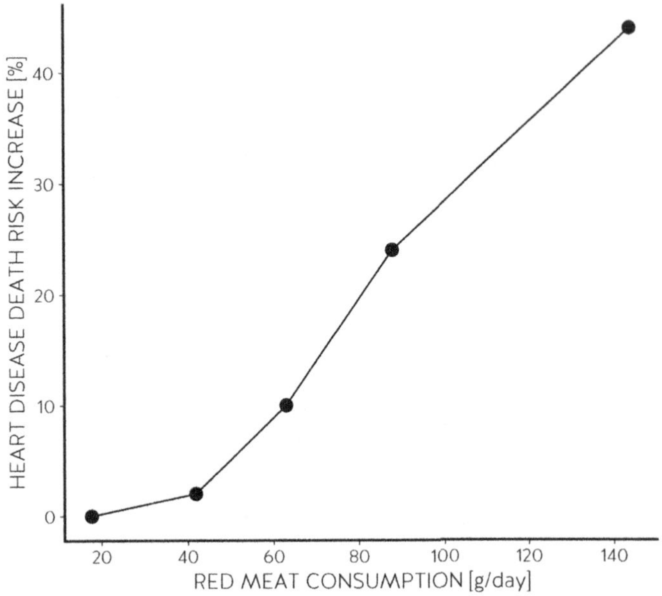

FUN FACT
Meats that are red when raw are defined as red meats. These include lamb, beef, and pork.

KEY TAKEAWAY
Limit the red meat consumption to 1/2 lb (280 g) or less per week to minimize the heart disease death risk.

- Red meat consumption increases the risk of perishing from cardiovascular disease.
- Those eating 140 grams of red meat per day have 44% higher death risk from heart disease compared to those eating just 20 grams of meat per day.
- The lowest risk is achieved by limiting meat intake to 40 grams per day. This translates to 280 grams (about 1/2 pound) of red meat per week.

R. Sinha, A. J. Cross, B. I. Graubard, M. F. Leitzmann, and A. Schatzkin, "Meat intake and mortality: a prospective study of over half a million people," Archives of Internal Medicine 169, No. 6 (2009): 562-571.

LOW CARB/HIGH PROTEIN DIETS INCREASE HEART DISEASE RISK

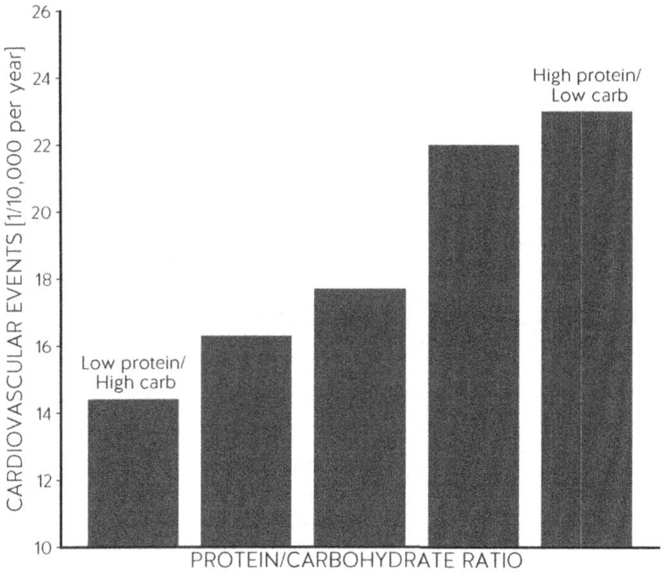

- Low carbohydrate diets are popular for weight management but diets high in animal protein are not optimal for heart health.
- Low carbohydrate/high *animal* protein diets are associated with increased risk of cardiovascular disease and stroke.
- In contrast, diets low in carbohydrates but high in *plant* protein and fats are healthy.

FUN FACT
Atkins diet and ketogenic diet are variations of the low-carb diet.

FUN FACT
The low-carb diet was first popularized by William Banting in 1863. Willams published a booklet "Letter on Corpulence Addressed to the Public", in which he described a diet for weight control giving up bread, butter, milk, sugar, beer, and potatoes.

KEY TAKEAWAY
Low carb/high animal protein diets increase heart disease risk. Low carb/high plant protein and fat diet is a healthier diet option.

P. Lagiou, S. Sandin, M. Lof, D. Trichopoulos, H.-O. Adami, and E. Weiderpass, "Low carbohydrate-high protein diet and incidence of cardiovascular diseases in Swedish women: prospective cohort study," BMJ: British Medical Journal 344 (2012): 1341-1345.

S. B. Seidelmann, B. Claggett, S. Cheng, M. Henglin, A. Shah, L. M. Steffen, A. R. Folsom, E. B. Rimm, W. C. Willett, and S. D. Solomon, "Dietary carbohydrate intake and mortality: a prospective cohort study and meta-analysis," The Lancet 3, No. 9 (2018): 419:428.

A MEAL WITH SATURATED FAT DRAMATICALLY AFFECTS BLOOD VESSELS

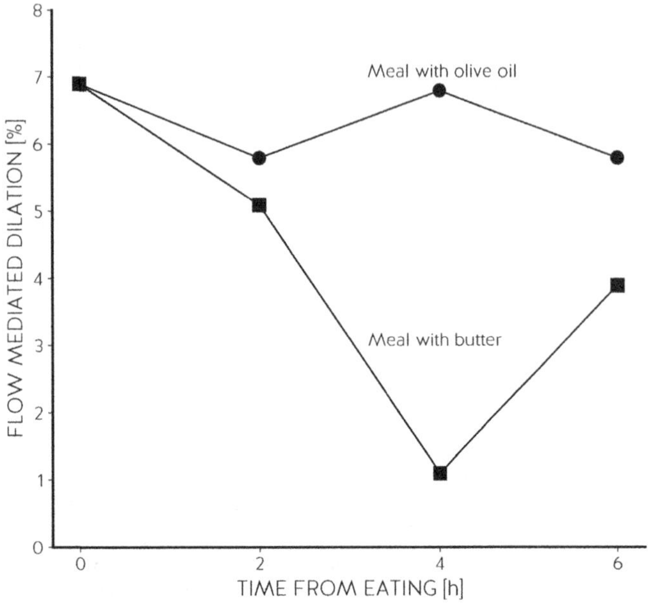

FUN FACT

Olive oil is approximately 13% saturated fat, 10% polyunsaturated fat, and 71% monounsaturated fat.

KEY TAKEAWAY

Saturated fat has an immediate negative effect on blood vessel functionality and blood lipid levels.

- The vascular activity after meals show dramatic differences depending on the type of digested fat.
- Meals containing saturated fat (butter) exerts a noxious effect on vascular functions that extends to 6 hours after dinner.
- Meal with mainly unsaturated fat (olive oil) did not deteriorate vascular activity.
- In addition, a meal with saturated fat (butter) increase the blood triglycerides level by more than 50%. No significant change is observed after the meal with unsaturated fat (olive oil).

N. Tentolouris, C. Arapostathi, D. Perrea, D. Kyriaki, C. Revenas, and N. Katsilambros, "Differential effects of two isoenergetic meals rich in saturated or monounsaturated fat on endothelial function in subjects with type 2 diabetes," Diabetes Care 31, No. 12 (2008): 2276–2278.

VASCULAR ACTIVITY DROPS AFTER EATING FAST FOOD

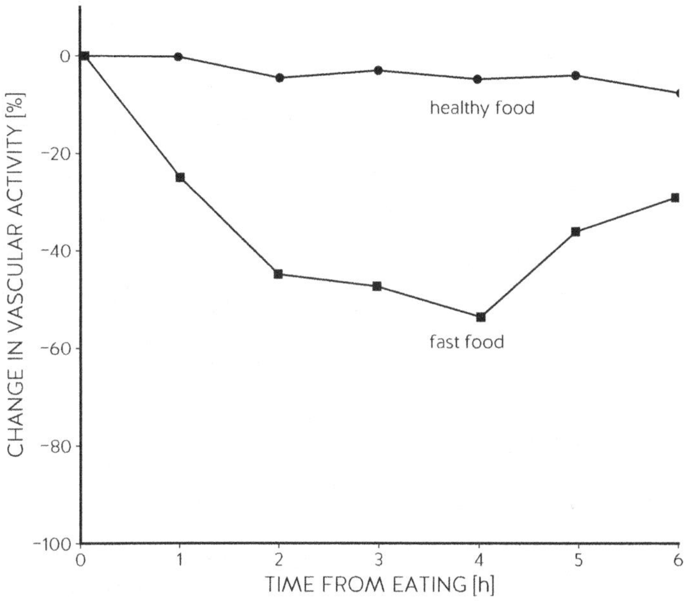

FUN FACT

A single fast food breakfast (Mc-Donalds Big Breakfast) has 18 g of saturated fat.

KEY TAKEAWAY

Feeling awful after eating fast food? There is scientific basis for it!

- A fast food breakfast has a dramatic negative effect on vascular activity defined as a change in artery diameter due to occlusion.
- Vascular activity drops by 50% after eating fast food and recovers only after 6 hours after breakfast.
- A low fat breakfast does not decrease vascular activity.

R. A. Vogel, M. C. Corretti, and G. D. Plotnick, "Effect of a single high-fat meal on endothelial function in healthy subjects," The American Journal of Cardiology 79, No. 3 (1997): 350-354.

HIGH-SALT MEALS IMPAIR BLOOD VESSELS

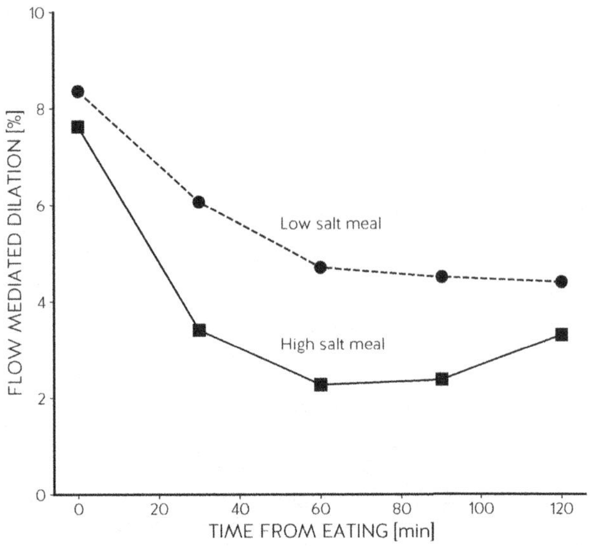

KEY TAKEAWAY

You already knew that too much salt is unhealthy. Negative effect on blood vessels is one more reason to avoid it.

- Saturated fats are not the only offender: a salty meal also has a dramatic and immediate negative effect on blood vessels.
- A high salt intake is also associated with high blood pressure which is a risk factor for heart disease.

K. M. Dickinson, P. M., Clifton, and J. B. Keogh, "Endothelial function is impaired after a high-salt meal in healthy subjects," The American Journal of Clinical Nutrition 93, No. 3 (2011): 500–505.

VINEGAR MAY IMPROVE CHOLESTEROL

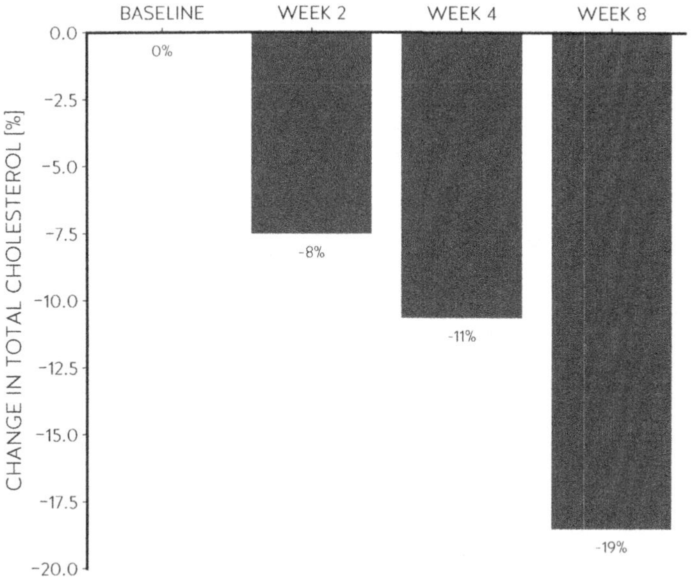

KEY TAKEAWAY

Vinegar may reduce cholesterol levels. Since it also helps in controlling blood glucose, it is a good idea to add vinegar to the diet for example in salad dressings.

- In a recent study, two tablespoons of apple cider vinegar twice a day significantly lowered total cholesterol.
- Both triglyceride and "bad cholesterol" (LDL) improved. "Good cholesterol" (HDL) was not affected.
- The study size was small and the diet was not controlled otherwise. More research is needed to confirm the findings.
- Vinegar also helps in improving post meal glucose levers (p. 81)

Z. Beheshti, Y. H. Chan, H. S. Nia, Hajihosseini, R. Nazari, and M. Shaabani, "Influence of apple cider vinegar on blood lipids," Life Science Journal 9, No. 4, (2012): 2431-2440.

CALORIE RESTRICTION IMPROVES HEART HEALTH MARKERS

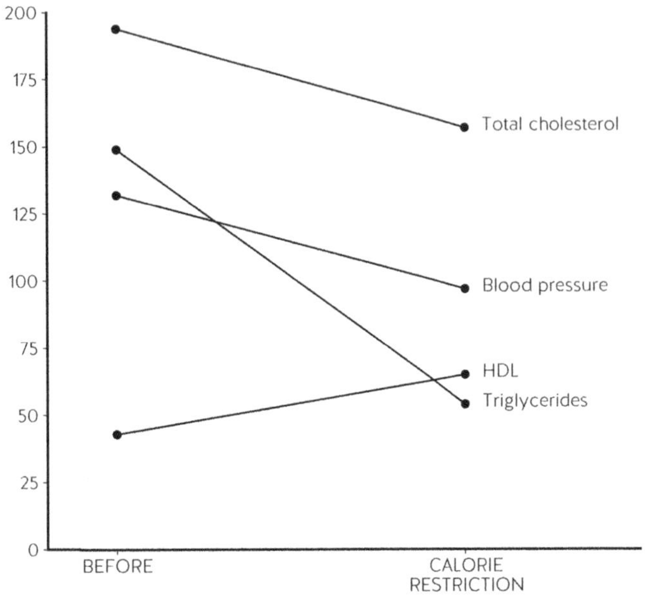

- Calorie restriction significantly improves cholesterol and blood pressure levels which are markers for cardiovascular health.
- Calorie restriction diet supplies more than 100% of the Recommended Daily Intake (RDI) for all of the essential nutrients, while minimizing energy content to less than 1,960 kcal/day which is below the recommended daily intake.
- Calorie restriction diet includes a wide variety of vegetables, fruits, nuts, dairy products, egg whites, wheat and soy proteins, and meat but strictly avoids processed foods and high glycemic foods (for example, refined carbohydrates, snacks, and soft drinks).

FUN FACT

Calorie restriction was popularized in 1980s by Dr. Walford who spend 2 years locked inside Biosphere 2 experiment. Due to problems in food production, the scientist inside Biosphere 2 were on a very low calorie diet but had excellent heart health markers.

KEY TAKEAWAY

Eating less than recommended daily calorie intake may not be for everyone but the positive effect on heart health make it a worthy consideration.

L. Fontana, T. E. Meyer, S. Klein, and J. O. Holloszy, "Long-term calorie restriction is highly effective in reducing the risk for atherosclerosis in humans," Proceedings of the National Academy of Sciences of the United States of America 101, No. 17 (2004): 6659-6663.

ALTERNATE DAY FASTING LOWERS CHOLESTEROL

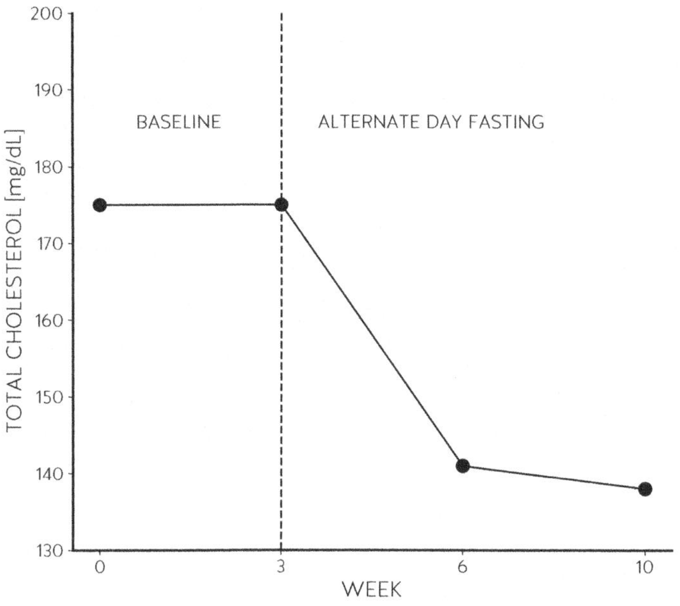

KEY TAKEAWAY
Fasting on alternate days may not be for everyone but the positive effect on heart health can be dramatic. Fasting intermittently 1-2 days every week may be an easier approach.

- Fasting on alternate days lowers cholesterol quickly and significantly.
- In just 3 weeks of alternate-day fasting, the total cholesterol dropped to below 150 mg/dL (3.9 mmol/L) where cardiovascular disease progression is thought to be arrested or even reversed.
- The "bad" LDL cholesterol and triacylglycerol levels are both reduced. The "good" HDL cholesterol is not affected by the alternate-day fasting.

K. A. Varady, S. Bhutani, E. C. Church, and M. C. Klempel, "Short-term modified alternate-day fasting: a novel dietary strategy for weight loss and cardioprotection in obese adults," The American Journal of Clinical Nutrition 90, No. 5 (2009): 1138-1143.

M. C. Klempel, C. M. Kroeger, K. A. Varady, "Alternate day fasting (ADF) with a high-fat diet produces similar weight loss and cardio-protection as ADF with a low-fat diet," Metabolism 62, No. 1 (2013): 137-143.

VITAMIN D DEFICIENCY INCREASES THE RISK OF DEATH FROM HEART DISEASE

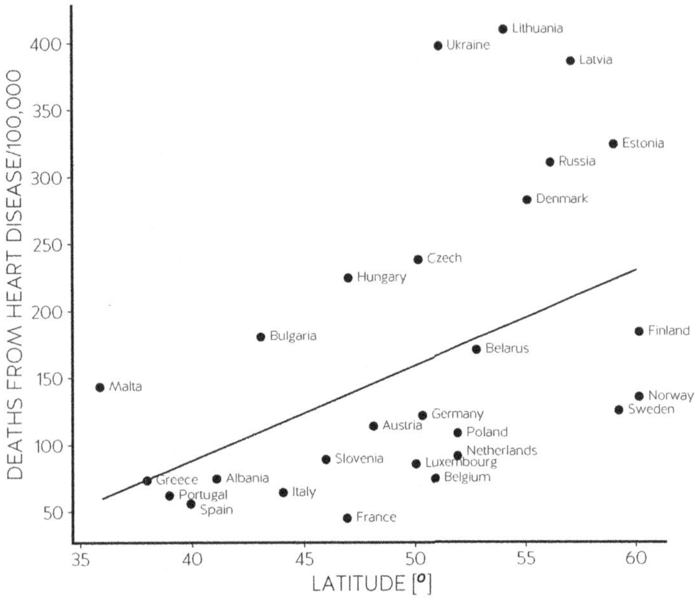

KEY TAKEAWAY

We have only recently started to appreciate the full importance of vitamin D on heart health. Vitamin D supplementation may decrease the risk of heart disease.

- Death rate from heart disease is higher in northern countries where solar radiation does not provide enough vitamin D.
- Death rate is also higher during winter months than summer months. Supplementing diet with vitamin D during winter, blunts the winter death peak.
- Vitamin D lowers C-reactive protein (CRP), which is a marker for inflammation and a risk factor for heart attacks.
- Vitamin D also protects against cancers (p. 97).

A. Zittermann, S. S. Schleithoff, and R. Koerfer, "Putting cardiovascular disease and vitamin D insufficiency into perspective," British Journal of Nutrition 94, No. 4, (2005): 483-492.

PROPER HYDRATION CAN REDUCE THE RISK OF DEATH FROM HEART DISEASE

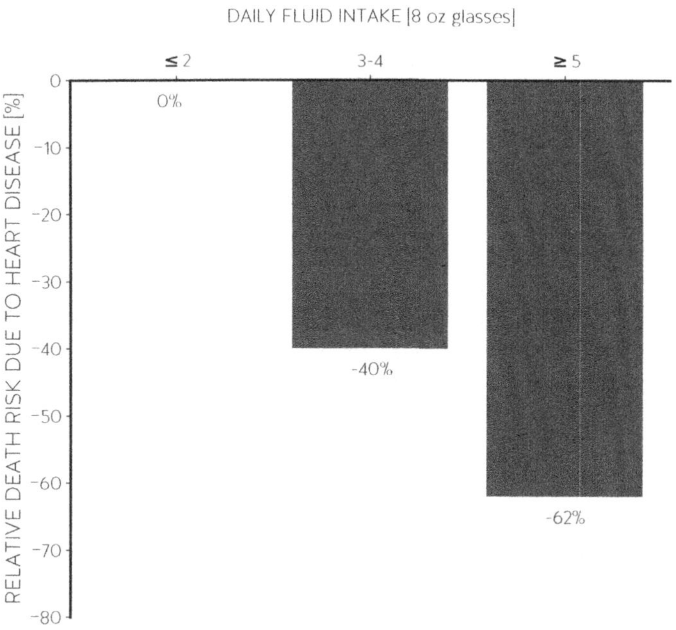

KEY TAKEAWAY
Drinking water is an easy, free, and remarkably effective way to reduce death risk.

- Insufficient water intake increases the risk of fatal heart disease.
- Drinking 5 or more glasses of liquids per day reduces the death risk by 62% compared to drinking just 2 glasses. One glass equals 8 oz (240 ml).
- Get a head start and start the day with a big glass of water!

J. Chan, S. F. Knutsen, G. G. Blix, J. W. Lee, and G. E. Fraser, "Water, other fluids, and fatal coronary heart disease: the Adventist Health Study," American Journal of Epidemiology 155, No. 9 (2002): 827-833.

ERECTILE DYSFUNCTION MAY BE DUE TO HEART DISEASE

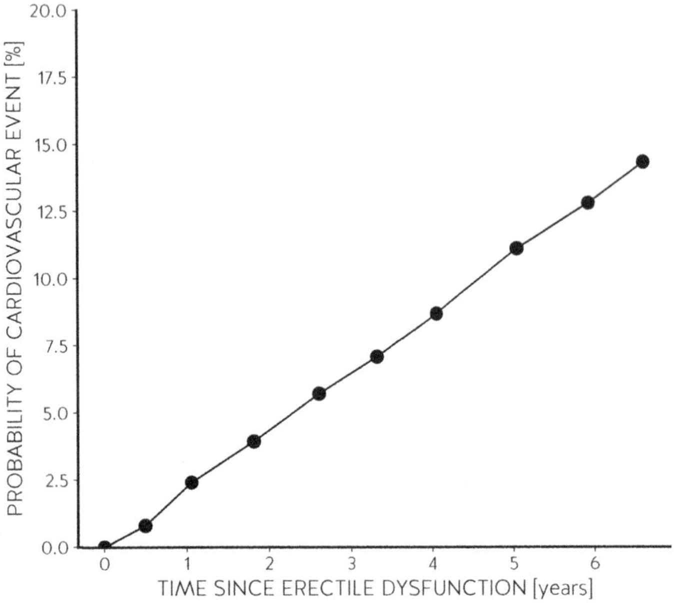

KEY TAKEAWAY
Heart health is connected to everything - including sex life.

- Erectile dysfunction may be an early marker for atherosclerosis and cardiovascular disease.
- After manifestation of erectile dysfunction, there is an 11% probability of a cardiovascular event such as a heart attack within 5 years.
- Conversely, avoiding heart disease and maintaining good blood flow to all parts of the body helps maintain erectile functions.

K. L. Billups, "Erectile dysfunction as an early sign of cardiovascular disease," International Journal of Impotence Research 17 (2005): S19.

I. M. Thompson, C. M. Tangen, P. J. Goodman, J. L. Probstfield, C. M. Moinpour, and C. A. Coltman, "Erectile dysfunction and subsequent cardiovascular disease," JAMA 294, No. 2 (2005): 2996-3002.

COFFEE CAN RAISE CHOLESTEROL

TYPE OF COFFEE PREPARATION TECHNIQUE		RISE IN CHOLESTEROL LEVEL WITH CONSUMPTION OF FIVE CUPS PER DAY [MG/DL]
Filtered	Boiled water is poured over finely-ground roasted coffee beans in a paper filter, either by hand or by using an electric coffee maker	0.0
Percolated	Coarsely-ground, roasted coffee beans are extracted by recirculating boiling water until the desired brew strength is reached	0.0
Instant	2-3g of soluble coffee granules are dissolved into 150-190 ml of hot water	0.4
Espresso	Hot water is forced under high pressure through a bed of finely ground, usually dark-roasted, coffee beans	3.9
Mocha	Just overheated water is forced through a bed of finely ground, usually dark-roasted, coffee beans	2.7
Boiled	Coarse grounds are boiled with water or infused with hot water ('infused' coffee), and the liquid is decanted without the use of a filter	7.4
Plunger pot ("French press")	Hot water is poured onto coarse grounds, and after 2-5 min the metal screen strainer is pushed down to separate the grounds from the fluid	9.0
Turkish/Greek	Very fine/powdery grounds are brought to a boil once or repeatedly, or incubated with hot water ('mud' coffee), and the liquid is decanted without the use of a filter	9.8

FUN FACT

The cholesterol-raising effect is due to oils left in coffee grounds. Don't drink the dreg in the bottom of your mug.

KEY TAKEAWAY

Oils in coffee can raise cholesterol. Drip coffee is safe as filtering eliminates the small coffee particles.

- Coffee oils can raise total and LDL cholesterol levels.
- Filtered coffee (drip coffee), percolated coffee, and instant coffee are free from cholesterol raising oils.

- Coffee prepared in a plunger pot (French press) or with the Turkish coffee method can raise cholesterol. Avoid drinking more than two cups per day.

R. Urgert and M. B. Katan, "The cholesterol-raising factor from coffee beans," Annual Review of Nutrition 17, No. 1 (2017): 305-324.

KEY TAKEAWAYS ON HEART DISEASE

Cardiovascular disease is a slowly progressing lifestyle disease that may be preventable with proper diet. Evidence shows that optimal cholesterol levels are less than 150 mg/dL (3.9 mmol/L) for total cholesterol and less than 70 mg/dL (1.7 mmol/L) for LDL cholesterol. LDL cholesterol cannot be too low.

A plant-based diet is the most effective way to maintain optimal cholesterol levels. Diets with animal products result in consistently higher cholesterol levels.

Other nutritional factors that help reduce cardiovascular disease risk are:

- Maintain an Omega6/Omega3 fat intake ratio between 1-3 by avoiding industrial vegetables oils. Instead, use oils that have Omega-3 fatty acid such as olive oil, avocado, or nut oils. In addition, you should supplement your diet with chia seeds, flax seeds, walnuts, or eat fish.
- Reduce red meat consumption to less than 0.5 lb (280 g) per week.
- Take B12 supplements or eat B12 fortified foods to help your body effectively remove toxic homocysteine.
- Avoid high-glycemic-index foods such as sugars, white bread, white rice, breakfast cereals, and white potato.
- Eat more fruit and vegetables.
- Eat a small amount of nuts daily. A small handful is enough.
- Obtain sufficient vitamin D.
- Restrict calorie intake by fasting or adopting a lower calorie diet.
- Drink five 8 oz cups of water daily.

DIABETES

Type-2 diabetes is a killer: Long-term complications from high blood sugar include heart disease, strokes, blindness, kidney failure, and poor blood flow in the limbs that may lead to amputations. On average, type-2 diabetes cuts a full decade of life expectancy. Nobody wants to experience this; yet, type-2 diabetes incidences have increased markedly since 1960s in parallel with growing obesity rates.

Diabetes typically develops due to the interplay between blood sugar and the insulin hormone that controls blood sugar. When a person eats, and sugar (glucose) enters into the bloodstream, the body produces insulin. This insulin response is a signal to body cells to absorb the excess blood glucose, to be used for energy at later time or converted to fat. As the blood glucose is lowered, insulin levels drop and the process is reversed: Body cells release glucose to blood stream and start to use stored fat for energy.

Problems occur when a person too frequently eats foods that raise the blood glucose level. The insulin levels remain high throughout the day, excess energy is converted to fat for long-term storage. Over time, the cells become insulin resistant leading to even higher levels of insulin. The feedback mechanism that drives the development of insulin resistance is illustrated in Fig 3.

The insulin cycle feeds on itself:

- High levels of insulin cause body fat to build up.
- Body fat reduces insulin sensitivity as cells become insulin resistant.
- The body produces an even higher amount of insulin in an effort to control sugar levels.

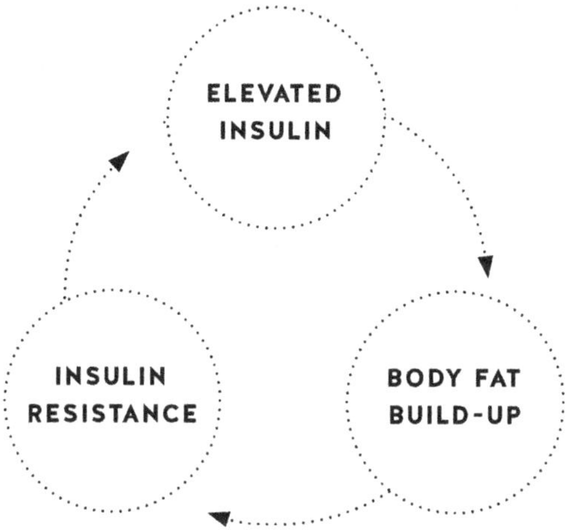

FIG 3. INSULIN FEEDBACK LOOP THAT LEADS TO INSULIN RESISTANCE

As the feedback cycle continues, the body starts to lose the ability to control blood sugar and fasting glucose levels become elevated. Eventually, the process can lead to full diabetes.

Part of the challenge with type-2 diabetes is that, like heart disease, it develops silently over decades. The good news is that diabetes is largely preventable and sometimes even reversible by disrupting the feedback cycle that leads to insulin resistance. When insulin levels are kept low, the body uses more of our stored energy reserves, body mass is reduced, and insulin sensitivity is improved. The fact that insulin resistance typically occurs in advance of impaired fasting glucose makes maintaining good insulin sensitivity critically important in our effort to avoid diabetes.

In this chapter, we cover risk factors for type-2 and how to minimize the risk of type-2 diabetes with a healthy diet.

24-HOUR INSULIN PROFILE IS ELEVATED FOR OBESE PEOPLE

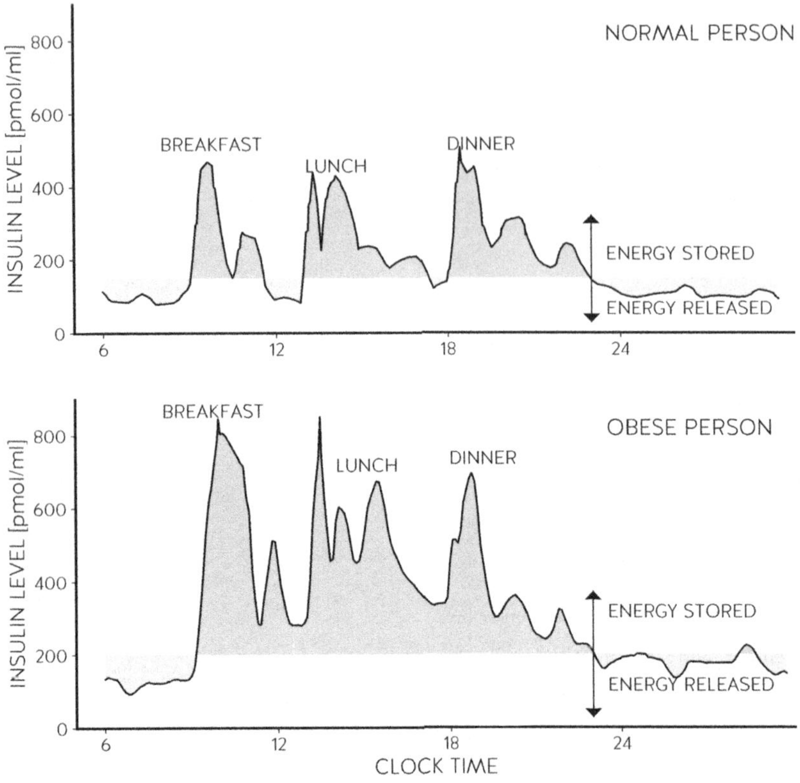

FUN FACT

Snacks are sometimes advertised as health promoting but there are no solid studies that support eating between meals. Too bad: "Lose 100 lb by snacking all the time" would be a bestselling book title.

KEY TAKEAWAY

Insulin spikes during a meal. The spikes are larger and longer for an obese person with lowered insulin sensitivity. Snacks between meals cause additional insulin spikes. A healthy snack is the one you skip.

- Insulin is a part of the human energy regulation system. Under normal conditions, high insulin levels encourage sugar and fat storage. Low insulin levels encourage the use of stored sugar and body fat.
- Normally, insulin spikes during a meal to signal the body to store the excess sugar. The insulin level drops between meals, which signals the body to release the stored energy.
- An obese person, defined as someone with a body mass index (BMI) over 30, has lowered insulin sensitivity. The obese person's insulin spikes higher and the insulin level

remains elevated between meals. The body is constantly in the energy-storage mode. This makes it very difficult to lower excess body weight.

- Over years, elevated levels of insulin may lead to insulin resistance or type-2 diabetes where the body is unresponsive to even high levels of insulin.
- Lower insulin levels and fewer insulin spikes help in avoiding weight gain and insulin resistance.
- Fasting between meals and healthy food choices help reduce insulin levels.

K. S. Polonsky, B. D. Given, and E. Van Cauter, "Twenty-four-hour profiles and pulsatile patterns of insulin secretion in normal and obese subjects," Journal of Clinical Investigation 81, No. 2 (1988): 442-448.

A. R. Saltiel, and C. R. Kahn, "Insulin signalling and the regulation of glucose and lipid metabolism," Nature 414 (2001): 799-806.

TYPE-2 DIABETES IS RARE ON PLANT-BASED DIETS

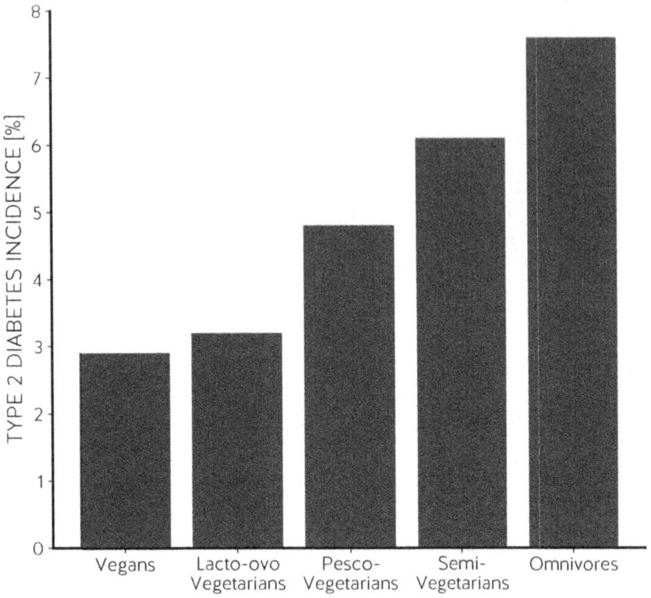

FUN FACT

According to the American Diabetes Association "it's best to limit your intake of red meat, which is often higher in saturated fat."

KEY TAKEAWAY

People who follow vegetarian and vegan diets have the lowest type-2 incidence rates.

- Type-2 diabetes incidence among vegans and lacto-ovo vegetarians is significantly lower than among omnivores (=meat eaters).

  Vegan diet includes only plants.

  Lacto-ovo vegetarian diet also includes dairy and eggs.

- Compared to vegans, pesco-vegetarians who consume fish, dairy products, and/or eggs have a higher rate of diabetes incidence.
- Semi-vegetarians who eat meat just once per week have a diabetes rate close to omnivores.

* There are multiple reasons why type-2 diabetes is more prevalent among people who eat meat and other animal products, including:

> Omnivores generally have higher body weight, which is a risk factor for diabetes.
>
> Eating animal protein also raises insulin levels and possibly contributes to insulin resistance.
>
> Vegetarian diets are rich in vegetables and fruits, foods that reduce oxidative stress and chronic inflammation.
>
> The vegetarian diet typically includes foods that have a low glycemic index such as beans, legumes, and nuts.

S. Tonstad, T. Butler, R. Yan, and G. E. Fraser, "Type of vegetarian diet, body weight, and prevalence of type-2 diabetes," Diabetes Care 32, No. 5 (2009): 791-796.

SATURATED FATS DECREASE INSULIN SENSITIVITY

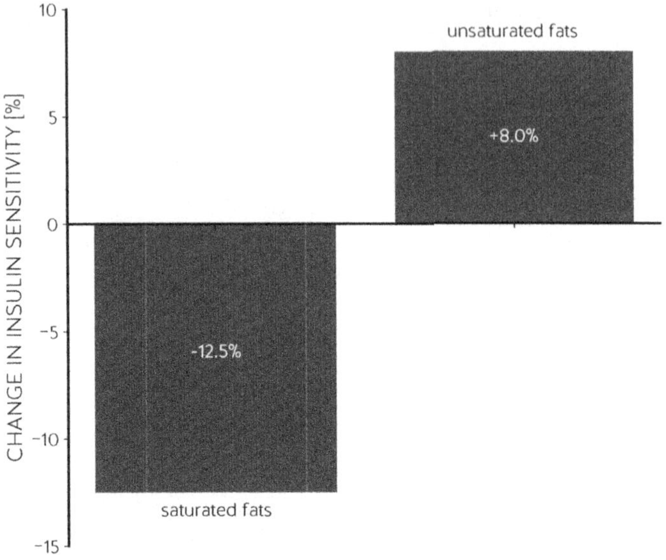

KEY TAKEAWAY
Saturated fats reduce and unsaturated fats improve insulin sensitivity.

- A diet high in saturated fats decreases insulin sensitivity in a clinical study.
- In contrast, a diet high in monounsaturated fats improves insulin sensitivity.
- The beneficial impact of the fat quality on insulin sensitivity is not seen in high-fat diets (>37% of energy from fats).

B. Vessby, M. Uusitupa, K. Hermansen, G. Riccardi, A. A. Rivellese, L. C. Tapsell, C. Nälsen, L. Berglund, A. Louheranta, B. M. Rasmussen, and G. D. Calvert, "Substituting dietary saturated for monounsaturated fat impairs insulin sensitivity in healthy men and women: The KANWU Study," Diabetologia 44, No. 3 (2001): 312-319.

ELEVATED FASTING GLUCOSE IS A SIGN OF INCREASED DIABETES RISK

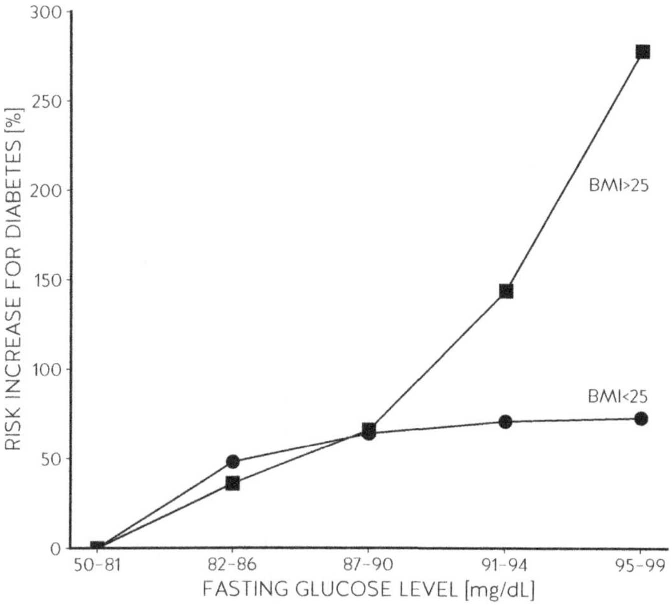

FUN FACT
Fasting glucose measurement is a cheap test typically done together with cholesterol measurement.

KEY TAKEAWAY
High fasting glucose is a risk factor for diabetes. High fasting glucose combined with overweight significantly increases the risk of type-2 diabetes.

- Fasting glucose test measures the amount of blood glucose after a 12-hour fast.
- Normal fasting glucose level was recently defined as less than 100 mg/dL (5.55 mmol/L) by the American Diabetes Association. Even the new, revised threshold may be too high. Glucose levels higher than 82 mg/dL (4.6 mmol/L) mark progressively increased risk of diabetes.
- Elevated fasting glucose levels combined with overweight (BMI>25) significantly increase the risk of type-2 diabetes.

A. Tirosh, I. Shai, D. Tekes-Manova, E. Israeli, D. Pereg, T. Shochat, and A. Rudich, "Normal fasting plasma glucose levels and type 2 diabetes in young men," New England Journal of Medicine 353, No. 14 (2005): 1454-1462.

J. V. Bjørnholt, G. Erikssen, E. Aaser, L. Sandvik, S. Nitter-Hauge, J. Jervell, J. Erikksen, and E. Thaulow, "Fasting blood glucose: an underestimated risk factor for cardiovascular death. Results from a 22-year follow-up of healthy nondiabetic men," Diabetes Care 22, No. 1 (1999): 45-49.

Caldwell B. Esselstyn, "Prevent and reverse heart disease: The revolutionary, scientifically proven, nutrition-based cure," Penguin, 2008.

ELEVATED HEMOGLOBIN A1C INCREASES DIABETES RISK

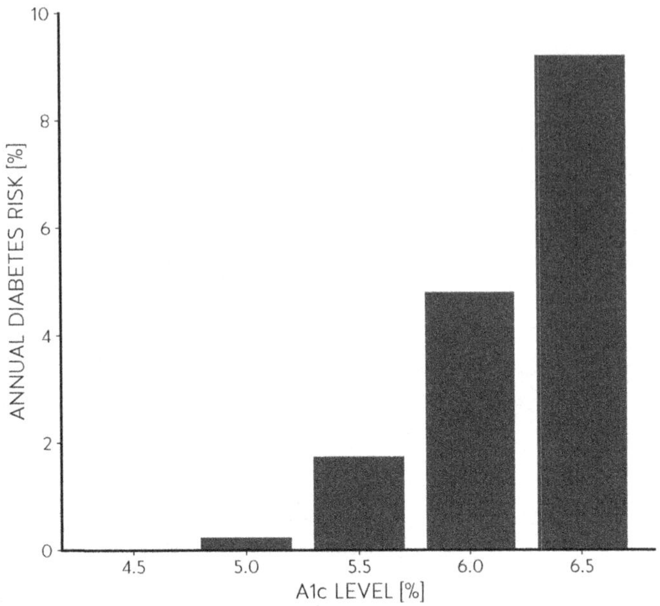

FUN FACT

A1c test is based on the attachment of glucose to hemoglobin in red blood cells. The red blood cells have the lifetime of 3-4 months and A1c measures average blood glucose level over this lifetime.

KEY TAKEAWAY

Hemoglobin A1c measures the average blood sugar level. Values higher than 5% mark a progressively increased risk of type-2 diabetes.

- The hemoglobin A1c test measures the average level of blood sugar over the past 2 to 3 months. The test is also called HbA1c. The test can be used to complement a fasting glucose test for diabetes screening and diagnosis.
- For people without diabetes, the normal range for the hemoglobin A1c level is between 4% and 5.6%. Ideally, hemoglobin A1c should be below 5% as this threshold marks a progressively increased risk of diabetes.

D. Edelman, M. K. Olsen, T. K. Dudley, A. C. Harris, and E. Z. Oddone, "Utility of hemoglobin A1c in predicting diabetes risk." Journal of General Internal Medicine 19, No. 12 (2004): 1175-1180.

X. Zhang, E. W. Gregg, D. F. Williamson, L. E. Barker, W. Thomas, K. McKeever Bullard, G. Imperatore, D. E. Williams, and A. L. Albright, "A1C level and future risk of diabetes: a systematic review," Diabetes Care 33, No. 7 (2010): 1665-1673.

HIGH GLYCEMIC INDEX FOODS INCREASE DIABETES RISK

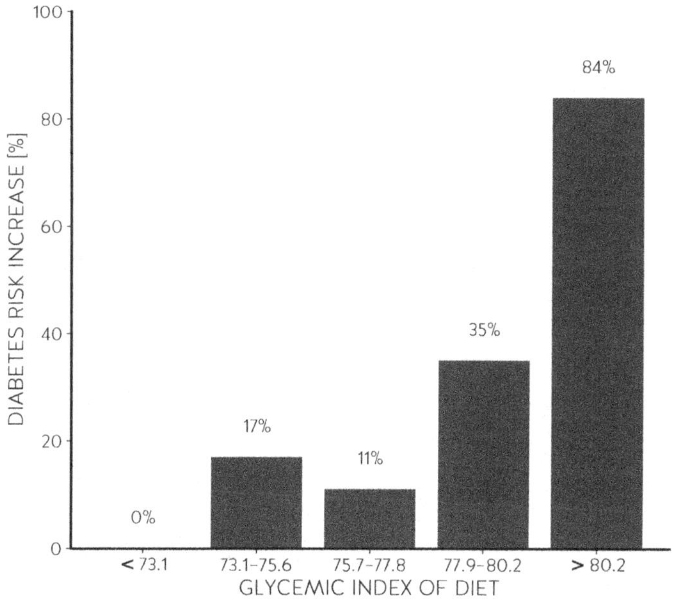

KEY TAKEAWAY

We all know that eating too much sugar is bad but one should also avoid eating other high glycemic index foods. These include refined carbohydrates such as white rice, pasta, and bread. Eating whole foods is good way to achieve a low glycemic index diet.

- Risk of diabetes increases with a high glycemic index diet. Diet with average glycemic index over 80 increases diabetes risk by 84%.
- High glycemic index foods (GI > 70) include glucose (dextrose, grape sugar), juices, sodas, high fructose corn syrup, white bread, white rice, corn flakes, and potatoes.
- Low glycemic index foods (GI < 55) include beans (black, pinto, kidney, lentil, peanut, chickpea), small seeds (sunflower, flax, pumpkin, poppy, sesame, hemp), walnuts, cashews, most whole intact grains (durum/spelt/kamut wheat, millet, oat, rye, rice, barley), most vegetables, most whole fruits (bananas, pineapple, peaches, strawberries, mangos), mushrooms, and chili peppers.

M. Schulze, B. Matthias, S. Liu, E. B. Rimm, J. E. Manson, W. C. Willett, and F. B. Hu, "Glycemic index, glycemic load, and dietary fiber intake and incidence of type 2 diabetes in younger and middle-aged women," The American Journal of Clinical Nutrition 80, No. 2 (2004): 348-356

INSULIN INDEX MAY BE A BETTER WAY TO RANK FOODS THAN GLYCEMIC INDEX

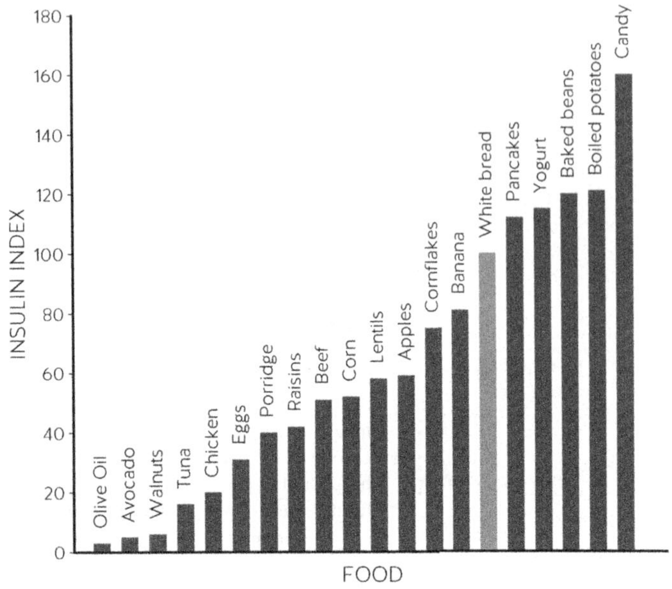

- The insulin index of a food represents how much a given food elevates insulin levels. White bread serves as the baseline with a score of 100.
- Sugary and starchy foods elicit high insulin responses due to the high carbohydrate content. These foods are best to be avoided as high levels of insulin may lead to insulin resistance.
- In general, all high glycemic index foods also have relatively high insulin index.
- Some foods, such as beef, raise insulin levels even though the glycemic index is low. Meat is harder on the human body than the glycemic index alone would suggest.
- Avocados and walnuts have low insulin index. They are great for snacks (although the best snack may be the skipped one).

FUN FACT

The Atkins diet is based on the idea of keeping the insulin level low by avoiding carbohydrates. Dr. Atkins used glycemic index as a proxy to determine which foods elicit high insulin response but this approach is not accurate. If Dr. Atkins had been aware of the insulin index, he might have recommended porridge instead of beef and dairy (yogurt).

KEY TAKEAWAY

Some foods raise insulin levels even though they are low in sugars and have a low glycemic index. It is best to moderate the consumption of high insulin index foods.

- A combination of foods can increase the insulin response. Milk spikes the insulin response. Fibrous foods (for example, vegetables, greens, and legumes) and berries lower insulin response.

K. J. Bell, R. Gray, D. Munns, P. Petocz, G. Howard, S. Colagiuri, and J. C. Brand-Miller, "Estimating insulin demand for protein-containing foods using the food insulin index," European Journal of Clinical Nutrition 68, No. 9 (2014): 1055-1059.

J. Bao, V. de Jong, F. Atkinson, P. Petocz, J. C. Brand-Miller, "Food insulin index: physiologic basis for predicting insulin demand evoked by composite meals," American Journal of Clinical Nutrition 90, No. 4 (2009): 986-992.

S. H. Holt, J. C. Miller, and P. Petocz, "An insulin index of foods: the insulin demand generated by 1000-kJ portions of common foods," American Journal of Clinical Nutrition 66, No. 5 (1997): 1264-1276.

BERRIES MODERATE BLOOD GLUCOSE

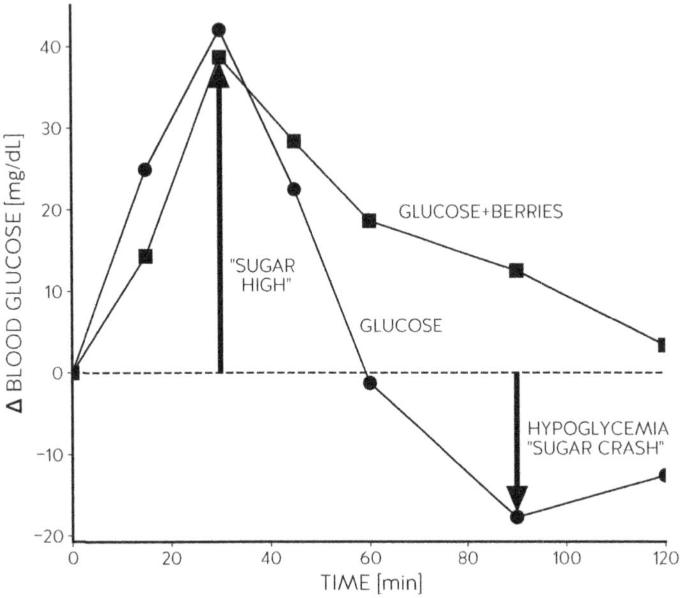

KEY TAKEAWAY

Eating berries have both short term and long term benefits: Berries slow the glucose absorption and improve insulin sensitivity.

- Eating pure sugar (glucose) leads to hypoglycemia or "sugar crash": 1. Blood glucose levels rise rapidly. 2. Body overcompensates by releasing too much insulin. 3. Glucose is absorbed by cells and glucose levels drop below the baseline level (hypoglycemia).
- Berries slow glucose absorption. The berries + glucose combination does not lead to hypoglycemia.
- Berries also have beneficial long term effects. Six weeks of consuming blueberry smoothies (yogurt, milk, and blueberry powder) twice daily improve insulin sensitivity in insulin resistant women and men.

R. Törrönen, M. Kolehmainen, E. Sarkkinen, H. Mykkänen, and L. Niskanen, "Postprandial glucose, insulin, and free fatty acid responses to sucrose consumed with blackcurrants and lingonberries in healthy women," The American Journal of Clinical Nutrition 96, No. 3 (2012): 527-533.

A. J. Stull, K. C. Cash, W. D. Johnson, C. M. Champagne, and W. T. Cefalu, "Bioactives in blueberries improve insulin sensitivity in obese, insulin-resistant men and women, The Journal of Nutrition 140, No. 10 (2010): 1764-1768.

EATING BERRIES LOWERS TYPE-2 DIABETES RISK

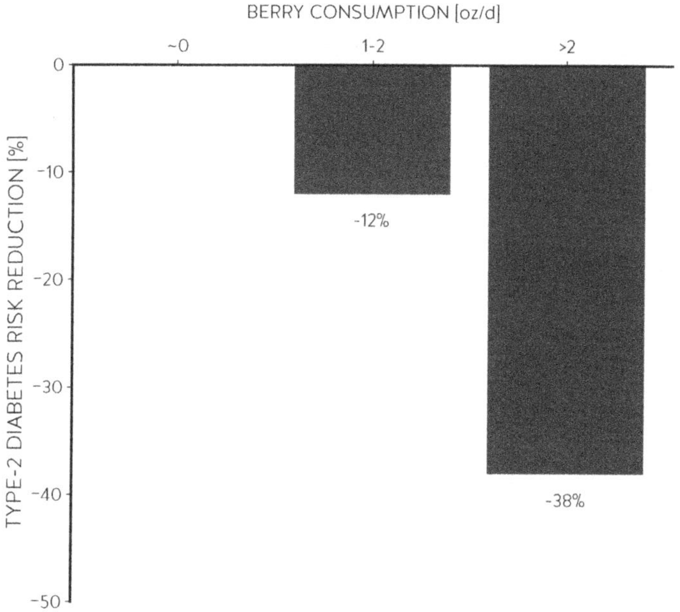

FUN FACT
2 oz (57 g) of berries is just about a handful.

KEY TAKEAWAY
Eating berries, fruits, and vegetables is a tasty way to lower diabetes risk.

- Eating more than 2 oz/day of berries lowers type-2 diabetes risk by 38%.
- Fruits and vegetables also lower type-2 diabetes risk. The biggest risk reduction is associated with the highest fruit and vegetable consumption.
- Fruit and berry juices do not offer similar benefits because the removal of fibers allows the sugars in juices to absorb too quickly and raise blood glucose levels.

J. Mursu, J. Virtanen, T.-P. Tuomainen, T. Nurmi, and S. Voutilainen, "Intake of fruit, berries, and vegetables and risk of type 2 diabetes in Finnish men: the Kuopio Ischaemic Heart Disease Risk Factor Study," The American Journal of Clinical Nutrition 99, No. 2 (2014): 328-333.

EATING NUTS LOWERS TYPE-2 DIABETES RISK

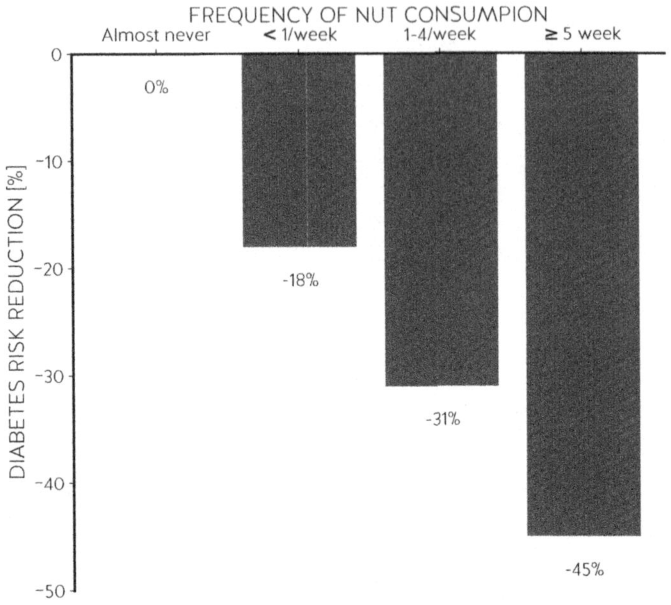

KEY TAKEAWAY
Eating nuts reduces type-2 diabetes risk.

- Nut consumption reduces type-2 diabetes risk. The risk reduction is seen even after adjusting for body mass, age, smoking, and other variables known to affect diabetes risk.
- Nuts are energy dense foods. To avoid increasing calorie intake, regular nut intake can be recommended as a replacement for refined grains or red or processed meats.

R. Jiang, J.A. E. Manson, M. J. Stampfer, S. Liu, W. C. Willett, and F. B. Hu, "Nut and peanut butter consumption and risk of type 2 diabetes in women," JAMA 288, No. 20 (2002): 2554-2560.

EATING FRUITS AND VEGETABLES LOWERS TYPE-2 DIABETES RISK

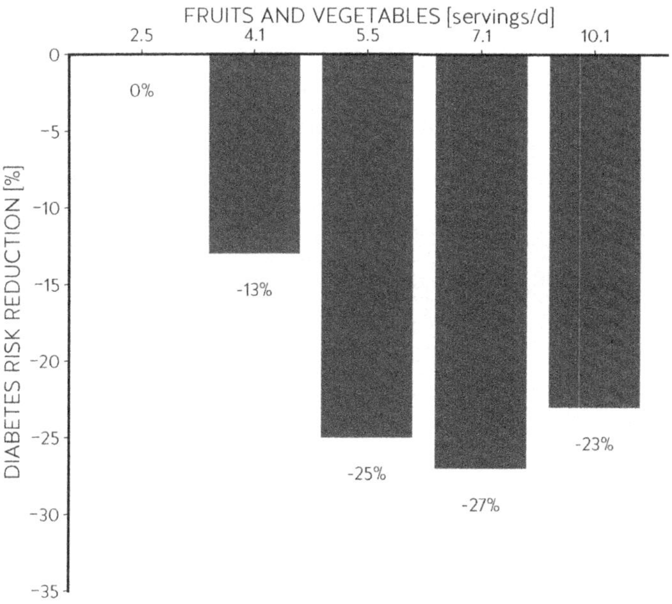

FUN FACT
Potatoes count as vegetable, however, in some studies potato consumption actually increases diabetes risk. This may be due to the fact that many potatoes are consumed as french fries which are often high on saturated fat and salt.

KEY TAKEAWAY
Eat plenty of fruits and vegetables to reduce diabetes risk.

- Eating fruits and vegetables reduces type-2 diabetes risk.

- The risk reduction is partially explained by associated reduction with other known risk factors. People eating lots of fruits and vegetables generally have lower calorie intake and have lower body weight.

- After adjusting for other risk factors, green leafy vegetables (spinach, kale, lettuce) and dark yellow vegetables (carrots, yellow squash, yams, sweet potatoes) may offer additional protection from diabetes.

S. Liu, M. Serdula, S.-J. Janket, N. R. Cook, H. D. Sesso, W. C. Willett, J.A. E. Manson, and J. E. Buring, "A prospective study of fruit and vegetable intake and the risk of type-2 diabetes in women," Diabetes Care 27, No. 12 (2004): 2993-2996.

MEAT INCREASES DIABETES RISK

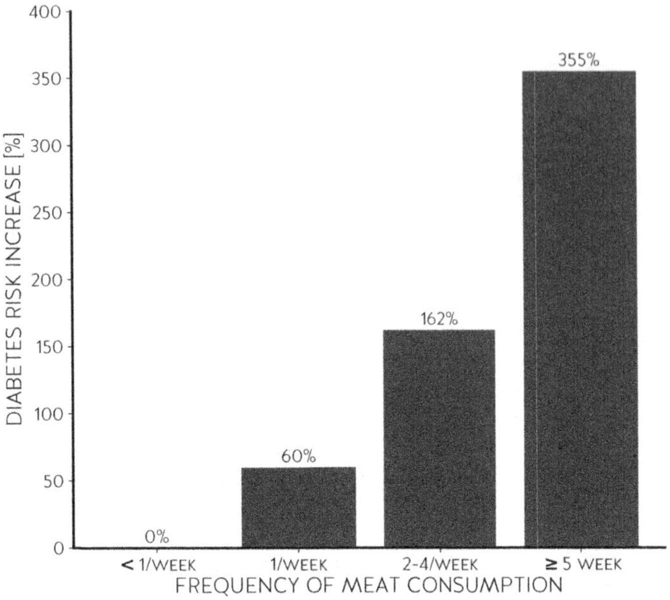

KEY TAKEAWAY
Frequent meat consumption significantly increases type-2 diabetes risk.

- Meat consumption increases type-2 diabetes risk. Those eating meat more than 5 times per week are 355% more likely to be diagnosed with type-2 diabetes than those eating meat less than 1 time per week.
- Part of the risk increase is due to difference in body mass. Meat eaters tend to have more fat than vegetarians.
- The risk increase, however, holds even after adjusting for known diabetes risk factors. There is some nutritional component in meats that increases diabetes risk.

M. B. Schulze, J. E. Manson, W. C. Willett, and F. B. Hu, "Processed meat intake and incidence of type 2 diabetes in younger and middle-aged women," Diabetologia 46, No. 11 (2003): 1465-1473.

T. T. Fung, M. Schulze, J. E. Manson, W. C. Willett, and F. B. Hu, "Dietary patterns, meat intake, and the risk of type 2 diabetes in women," Archives of Internal Medicine 164, No. 20 (2004): 2235-2240.

INSULIN RESPONSE INCREASES WITH COMBINATION OF SUGAR + BEEF

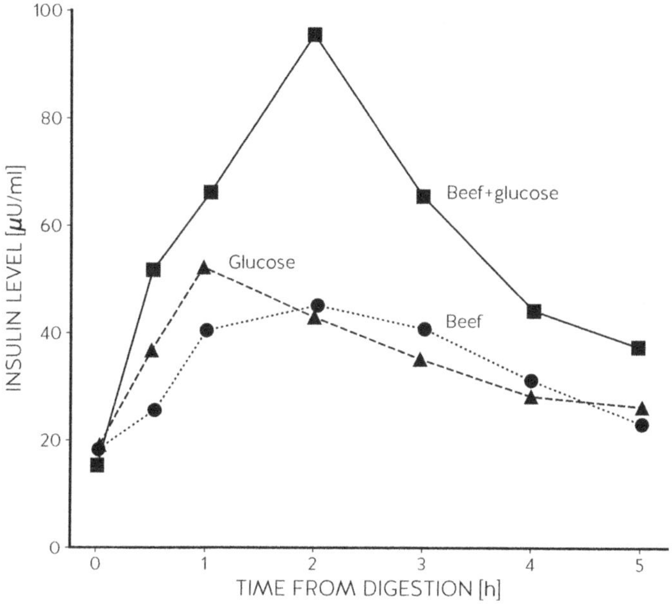

FUN FACT

A typical fast food meal of hamburger and soda is a perfect-storm combination of beef and sugar.

KEY TAKEAWAY

Sugar and meat together spikes insulin levels. Eating fast food meals (hamburger meat + soda) regularly can contribute to the development of insulin resistance, obesity, and type-2 diabetes.

- Combinations of foods may increase insulin response.
- Eating sugars (glucose) and hamburger meat together increases insulin response.
- Frequent elevated insulin spikes from sugar and beef combination can lead to the insulin resistance.

F. Nuttall, A. Mooradian, M. Gannon, C. Billington, and P: Krezowski, "Effect of protein ingestion on the glucose and insulin response to a standardized oral glucose load," Diabetes Care 7, No. 5 (1984): 465-470.

INSULIN RESPONSE IS SPIKED BY MILK

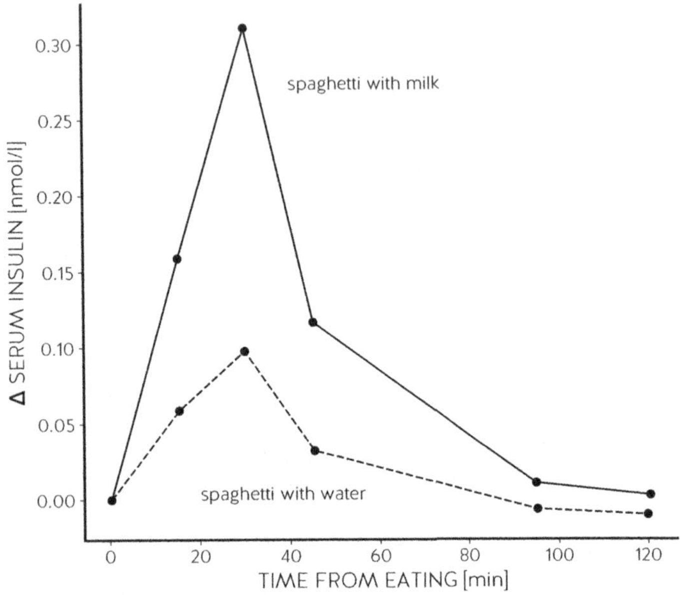

KEY TAKEAWAY

To avoid excessive insulin spikes, it is better to drink water than milk with meals.

- Combination of milk and pasta increases insulin levels compared to pasta with water.
- Increased insulin is undesirable because high insulin levels can decrease insulin sensitivity, which may lead to diabetes.

H. Elmstahl Liljeberg, and I. Bjorck, "Milk as a supplement to mixed meals may elevate postprandial insulinaemia," European Journal of Clinical Nutrition 55, No. 11 (2001): 994-999.

VINEGAR IMPROVES GLUCOSE AND INSULIN RESPONSE

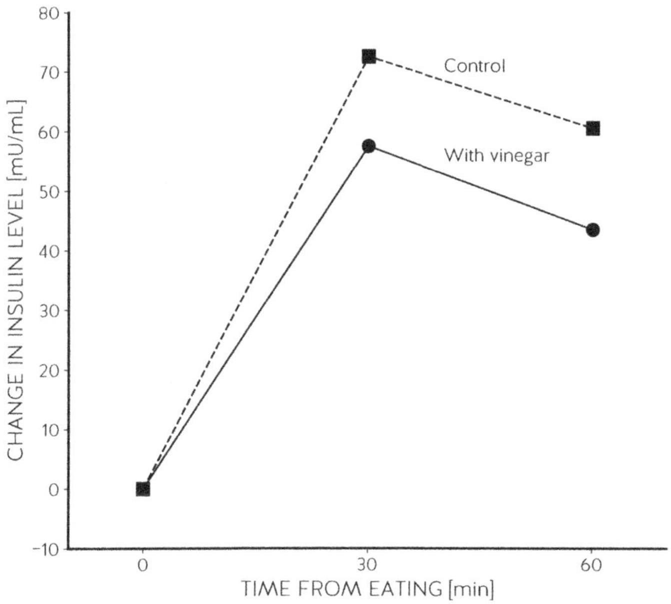

- A tablespoon of apple cider vinegar taken before a starchy meal improves glucose and insulin response. Both glucose and insulin levels are lower with vinegar consumption.
- Consistent vinegar use before meals may be more effective in reducing fasting blood glucose concentrations than popular type-2 diabetes medications such as metformin and rosiglitazone.

FUN FACT

Adding vinegar to starchy foods is a common practice in different cultures. For example, Japanese traditionally add vinegar to sushi rice, British add vinegar to fish and chips (potatoes), and Mediterranean cultures dip bread in olive oil and vinegar.

KEY TAKEAWAY

Consume vinegar before or during a starchy meal. Alternatively, add vinegar to a starchy meal.

C. S. Johnston, C. M. Kim, and A. J. Buller, "Vinegar improves insulin sensitivity to a high-carbohydrate meal in subjects with insulin resistance or type 2 diabetes," Diabetes Care 27, No. 1 (2004): 281-282.

F. Shishehbor, A. Mansoori, and F. Shirani, "Vinegar consumption can attenuate postprandial glucose and insulin responses; a systematic review and meta-analysis of clinical trials," Diabetes Research and Clinical Practice 127, (2017): 1-9.

C. S. Johnston, S. Quagliano, and S. White, "Vinegar ingestion at mealtime reduced fasting blood glucose concentrations in healthy adults at risk for type 2 diabetes," Journal of Functional Foods 5, No. 4 (2013): 2007-2011.

LOWERING BODY MASS INDEX (BMI) IMPROVES FASTING GLUCOSE

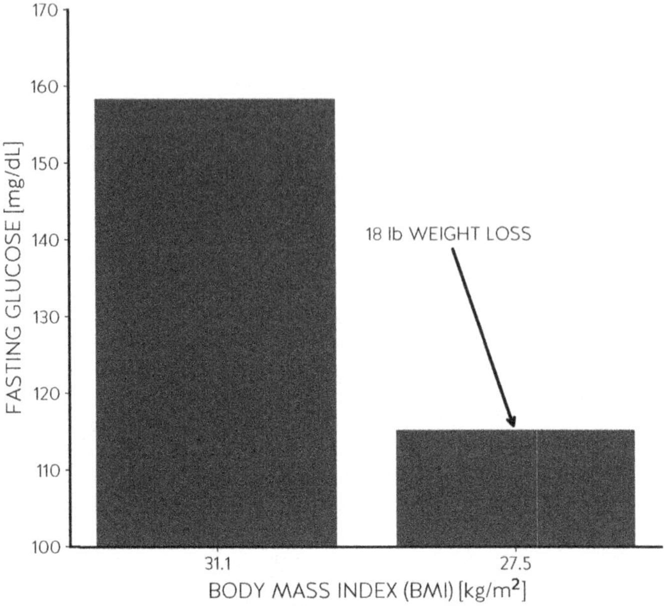

KEY TAKEAWAY
Lowering body weight is the most effective way to improve fasting glucose and insulin sensitivity.

- Lowering body weight can reverse type-2 diabetes.
- A modest 18 lb weight reduction in obese patients with type-2 diabetes lowered the average fasting glucose from 158 mg/dL (8.8 mmol/L) to 115 mg/dL (6.4 mmol/L), and the average insulin response dropped by 62%.
- Weight reduction also improved lipid levels. The average LDL cholesterol dropped from 119 mg/dL to 102 mg/dL (from 3.1 mmol/L to 2.6 mmol/L).

K. F. Petersen, S. Dufour, D. Befroy, M. Lehrke, R. E. Hendler, and G. I. Shulman, "Reversal of nonalcoholic hepatic steatosis, hepatic insulin resistance, and hyperglycemia by moderate weight reduction in patients with type-2 diabetes," Diabetes 54, No. 3 (2005): 603-608.

FASTING LOWERS INSULIN LEVELS

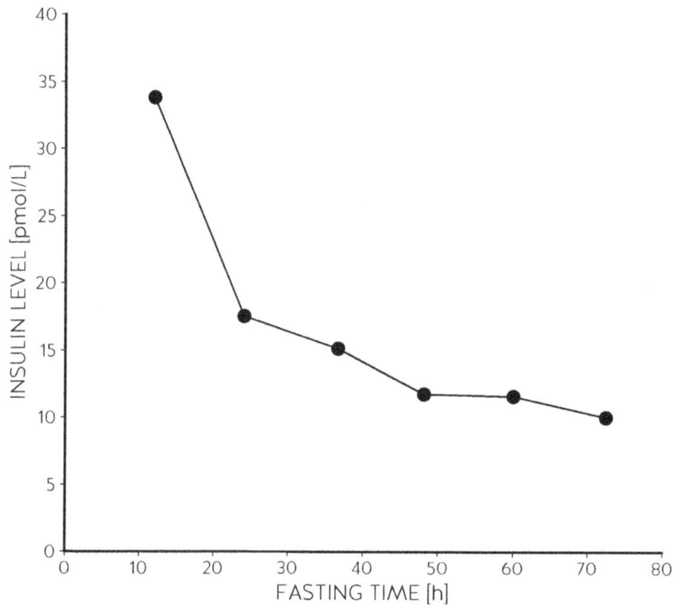

KEY TAKEAWAY
Fasting periodically for up to 24 hours is an effective way to reduce type-2 diabetes risk factors.

- Blood insulin levels drop while fasting. This transitions the body to use stored fat reserves.
- Even relatively short fasts are beneficial. In clinical trials, alternate-day fasting is shown to increase insulin sensitivity and lower body fat.

S. R. Stannard, M. W. Thompson, K. Fairbairn, B. Huard, T. Sachinwalla, and C. H. Thompson, "Fasting for 72 h increases intramyocellular lipid content in nondiabetic, physically fit men," American Journal of Physiology-Endocrinology and Metabolism 283, No. 6 (2002): E1185-E1191.

K. A. Varady, M. K. Hellerstein, "Alternate-day fasting and chronic disease prevention: a review of human and animal trials," The American Journal of Clinical Nutrition, 86, No. 1 (2007): 7-13.

N. Halberg, M. Henriksen, N. Söderhamn, B. Stallknecht, T. Ploug, P. Schjerling, and F. Dela, "Effect of intermittent fasting and refeeding on insulin action in healthy men," Journal of Applied Physiology 99, No. 6 (2005): 2128-2136.

KEY TAKEAWAYS ON DIABETES

Type-2 diabetes is a largely preventable lifestyle disease. The key to preventing diabetes is to have good insulin sensitivity by maintaining low body fat, eating low glycemic index foods, and reducing meat and saturated fat intake. In addition, fasting is a very effective way to lower insulin levels, improve insulin sensitivity, and reduce body weight. Overweight and obesity are the biggest risk factors for diabetes. Maintaining normal body weight is the most effective way to reduce the risk of diabetes.

Certain foods, such as berries and vinegar, lower blood glucose and insulin, which helps to lower type-2 diabetes risk. Some foods, such as beef, increase the insulin levels more than the glycemic index suggests. The combination of certain foods, such as sugar and beef or milk and pasta, elicit even higher insulin spikes. More research is needed, but it may be better to drink water rather than sugary drinks or milk with meals.

CANCER

Cancer is a truly scary disease where normal cells mutate into abnormal cells that grow quickly and lack normal cell death. While some cancers are treatable, many forms of cancers eventually cause death. The good news is that many cancers are preventable by avoiding excess body weight and eating right.

Is this chapter, we dive into the relationship between cancer and diet to learn which foods contribute to cancer and which foods can help protect us from cancer.

DIET AND OBESITY CAUSE MOST CANCERS

ENVIROMENTAL NON-TOBACCO CAUSES OF CANCER

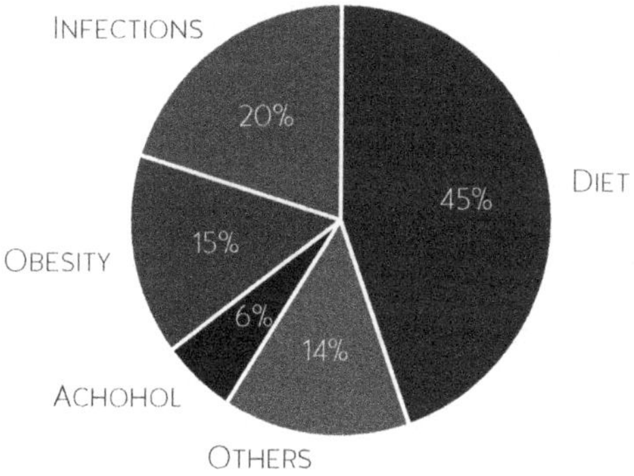

NOT FUN FACT

In 70s, the 5-year survival rate for people diagnosed with cancer was 49%. Today, it is 69%. Cancer prevention is easier than curing the cancer.

KEY TAKEAWAY

Healthy diet cannot eliminate all cancers but eating healthily can reduce the cancer risk by 30-60%.

- Only 5-10% of cancers are due to genetic factors while 90-95% of cancers are due to environmental factors. This makes cancer a largely preventable disease.
- For non-smokers, the controllable environmental factors are diet, body weight, and alcohol consumption. In total, these account for over half of all cancers.

P. Anand, B. A. Kunnumakara, C. Sundaram, K. B. Harikumar, S. T. Tharakan, O. S. Lai, B. Sung, and B. B. Aggarwal, "Cancer is a preventable disease that requires major lifestyle changes," Pharmaceutical Research 25, No. 9 (2008): 2097-2116.

L. H. Kushi, T. Byers, C. Doyle, E. V. Bandera, M. McCullough, T. Gansler, K. S. Andrews, and M. J. Thun, "American cancer society guidelines on nutrition and physical activity for cancer prevention: reducing the risk of cancer with healthy food choices and physical activity," CA: A Cancer Journal for Clinicians 56, No. 5 (2006): 254-281.

MEAT CONSUMPTION INCREASES CANCER RISK

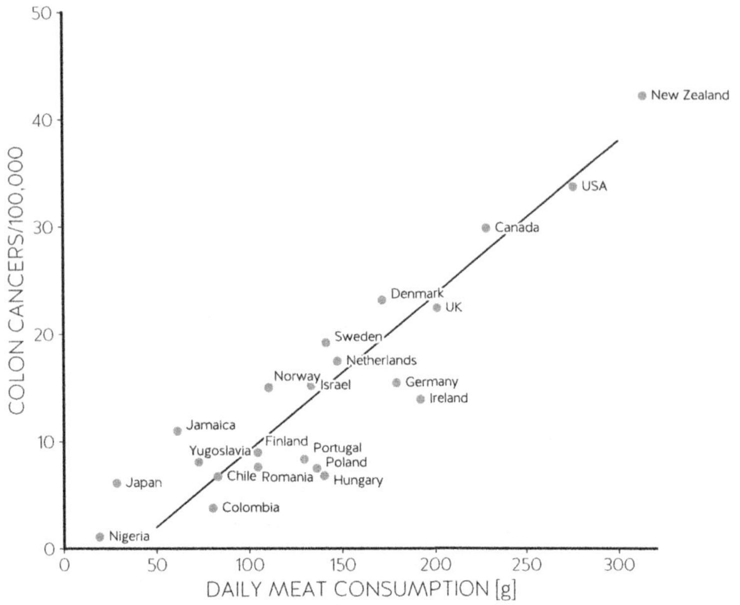

- Gastro-Intestinal (GI) cancers affect the digestive system. This includes the liver, pancreas, stomach, small intestine, and bowel.
- GI cancers are the most common form of cancer and are responsible for more deaths than any other form of cancer.
- GI cancer is strongly linked to meat consumption. GI cancer is most common in the USA and New Zealand where meat consumption is high. Conversely, it is rare in Nigeria and Japan where meat consumption is low.
- To minimize cancer risk, limit red meat consumption to less than 250 grams a week (less than 1/2 pound per week).

FUN FACT

There is convincing evidence that processed meats cause cancer. The World Health Organization (WHO) classifies processed meat as a Group 1 carcinogen.

KEY TAKEAWAY

Red meat consumption, especially of processed red meat like bacon, sausage, and hot dogs, is associated with GI cancers. Avoid all processed meats and limit the consumption of red meat.

- Evidence on white meats such as chicken is mixed. People who eat white meats have a higher prevalence of cancers than vegetarians but conclusive evidence on causal link is lacking. However, while white meats may not directly cause cancers, unlike fruits and vegetables, they do not protect from cancers. It is best to eat all meats in moderation.

B. Armstrong and R. Doll, "Environmental factors and cancer incidence and mortality in different countries, with special reference to dietary practices," International Journal of Cancer 15, No. 4 (1975): 617-631.

World Cancer Research Fund, and American Institute for Cancer Research, "Food, nutrition, physical activity, and the prevention of cancer: a global perspective, Continuous Update Project," (2018), available at http://www.dietandcancerreport.org/

ALCOHOL INCREASES CANCER RISK

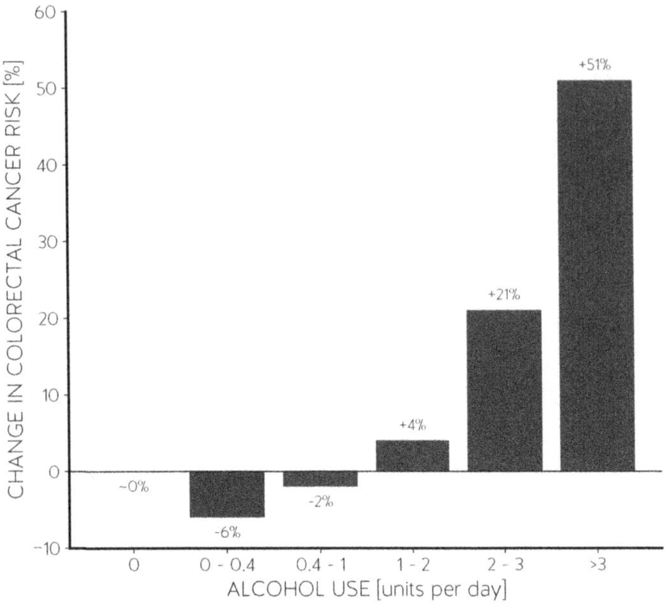

FUN FACT
The World Health Organization (WHO) classifies alcohol (ethanol) as Group 1 carcinogen.

FUN FACT
One unit of alcohol, or a standard drink, contains 14 g of pure alcohol as found in:
- 12 ounces (350 ml) of regular beer, which is 5% alcohol
- 5 ounces (150 ml) of wine, which is 12% alcohol
- 1.5 ounces (44 ml) of distilled spirits, which is 40% alcohol

KEY TAKEAWAY
Alcohol is a cancer causing substance. Limiting consumption to 1 unit or less per day minimizes the cancer risk.

- Consuming small amounts of alcohol may be enjoyable and might confer some health benefits: Drinking less than one unit per day may reduce colorectal cancer risk.
- Drinking more than one unit per day increases colorectal cancer risk.
- A significant risk increase occurs when consuming more than three units per day.
- Alcohol use also increases the risk of other types of cancers. For instance, drinking more than two units per day increases breast cancer risk by 20%.

E. Cho, S. A. Smith-Warner, J. Ritz, P. A. Van Den Brandt, G. A. Colditz, A. R. Folsom, J. L. Freudenheim, E. Giovannucci, R. A. Goldbohm, S. Graham, and L. Holmberg, "Alcohol intake and colorectal cancer: a pooled analysis of 8 cohort studies," Annals of Internal Medicine 140, No. 8 (2004): 603-613.

P. Boyle and P. Boffetta, "Alcohol consumption and breast cancer risk," Breast Cancer Research 11, No. 3 (2009): S3.

LOW BODY MASS INDEX (BMI) MINIMIZES CANCER RISK

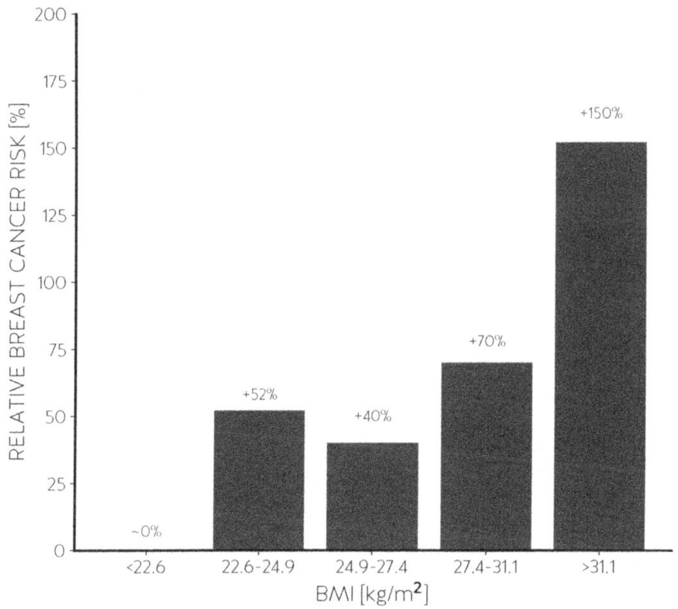

FUN FACT

In the last 50 years, the obesity rate has more than tripled from 12% to 50% in USA, negating some of the medical advances in cancer care. More than two out of three adults are overweight or are obese.

KEY TAKEAWAY

Being overweight significantly increases cancer risk.

- Cancer risk increases with an increase in body mass index (BMI). People with a BMI > 30 kg/m^2 have 150% higher breast cancer risk than those with a BMI < 22.6 kg/m^2.
- Similar trends are seen for many other types of cancers. For example, a BMI > 30 kg/m^2 increases colon cancer risk by 140% among 55-79 year-old adults.
- Obesity is identified as the single biggest risk factor for cancer.
- Cancer risk is the lowest for people in the lower end of the normal BMI range of 20-25 kg/m^2.

L. M. Morimoto et al., "Obesity, body size, and risk of postmenopausal breast cancer: the Women's Health Initiative (United States)," Cancer Causes & Control 13, No. 8 (2002): 741-751.

L. L. Moore, M. L. Bradlee, M. R. Singer, G. L. Splansky, M. H. Proctor, R. C. Ellison, and B. E. Kreger, "BMI and waist circumference as predictors of lifetime colon cancer risk in Framingham Study adults," International Journal of Obesity 28, No. 4 (2004): 559-567.

HIGH GLYCEMIC INDEX DIET INCREASES CANCER RISK

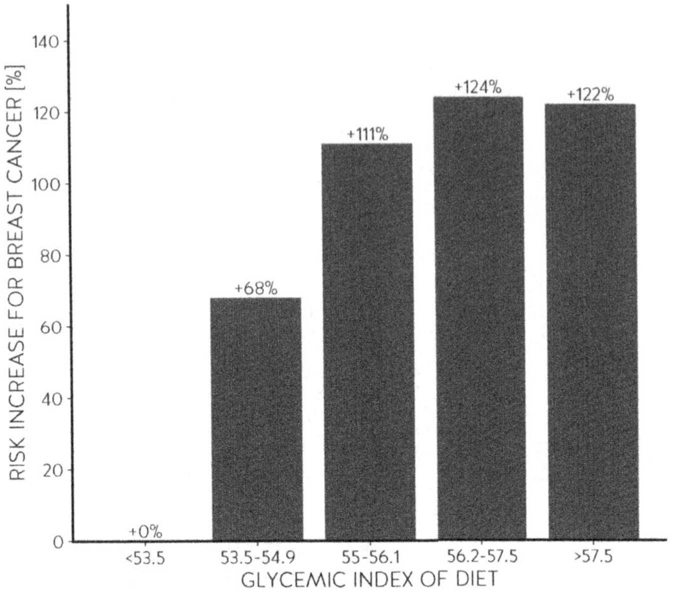

FUN FACT

The elevated uptake of glucose characterizes the majority of cancers, which explains why a diet that raises blood glucose is conductive to cancer growth.

KEY TAKEAWAY

Avoid sugary and starchy foods to help avoid cancer. Instead, eat whole foods and plants.

- Glycemic index of diet correlates with breast cancer rate. A diet with a high glycemic index increases breast cancer risk by >100% compared to diets with the lowest glycemic index.
- Even diets with a moderate glycemic index show an increased cancer rate.
- Avoid sugary foods and processed foods.
- Plants, nuts, and whole grains have a low glycemic index. These foods should form the majority of the diet.

S. Sieri, V. Pala, F. Brighenti, N. Pellegrini, P. Muti, A. Micheli, A. Evangelista, S. Grioni, P. Contiero, F. Berrino, V. and Krogh, "Dietary glycemic index, glycemic load, and the risk of breast cancer in an Italian prospective cohort study," The American Journal of Clinical Nutrition 86, No. 4, (2007): 1160-1166.

VEGETABLES DECREASE CANCER RISK

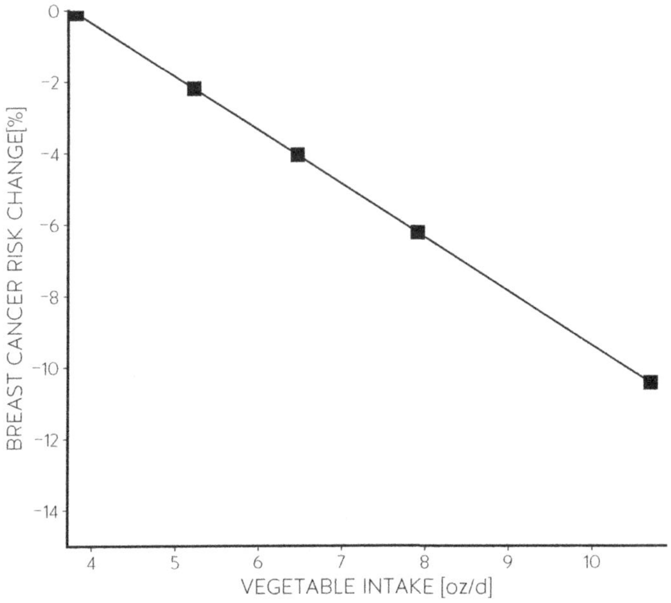

FUN FACT

The most popular vegetable in the United States is the potato followed by the tomato which is a rather sad fact since this is driven by consumption of french fries and pizza.

KEY TAKEAWAY

Everyone should eat multiple servings of vegetables every day to reduce cancer risk. The more, the better.

- Eating vegetables decreases the risk of breast cancer.
- Eating more vegetables also decrease the risk of other types of cancers. For example, increased vegetable consumption decreases colon, stomach, and prostate cancer risks.

D. T. Verhoeven, N. Assen, R. A. Goldbohm, E. Dorant, P. Van't Veer, F. Sturmans, R. J. Hermus, and P. A. Van den Brandt. "Vitamins C and E, retinol, beta-carotene and dietary fibre in relation to breast cancer risk: a prospective cohort study," British Journal of Cancer 75, No. 1 (1997): 149-155.

K. A. Steinmetz, L. H. Kushi, R. M. Bostick, A. R. Folsom, and J. D. Potter, "Vegetables, fruit, and colon cancer in the Iowa women's health study," American Journal of Epidemiology 139, No. 1 (1994): 1-15.

G. Block, B. Patterson, and A. Subar, "Fruit, vegetables, and cancer prevention: a review of the epidemiological evidence," Nutrition and Cancer 18, No. 1 (1992): 1-29.

FRUITS DECREASE CANCER RISK

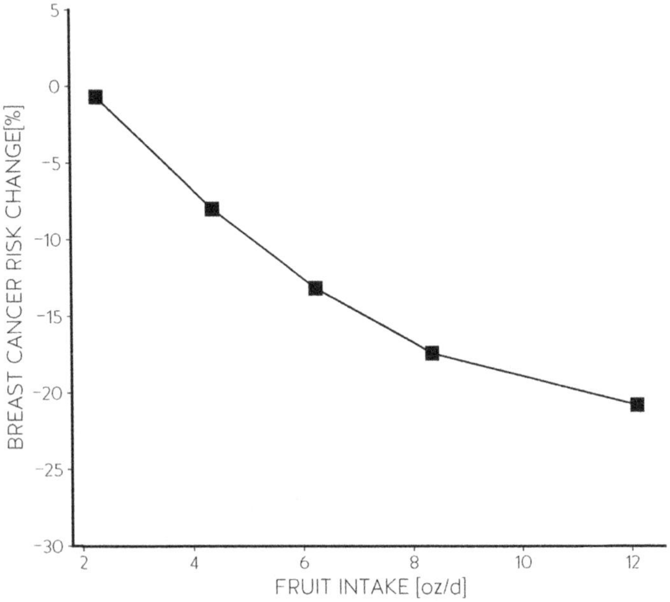

FUN FACT

Bananas and apples are neck to neck the most popular fruits in United States. On average person consumes over ten pounds of each per year.

KEY TAKEAWAY

Everyone should eat multiple servings of fruit every day to reduce cancer risk. The more, the better.

- Eating fruits decreases breast cancer risk.
- Eating more fruit also decreases the risk of other types of cancers. For example, fruit intake decreases colon, stomach, and prostate cancer risk.

D. T. Verhoeven, N. Assen, R. A. Goldbohm, E. Dorant, P. Van't Veer, F. Sturmans, R. J. Hermus, and P. A. Van den Brandt. "Vitamins C and E, retinol, beta-carotene and dietary fibre in relation to breast cancer risk: a prospective cohort study," British Journal of Cancer 75, No. 1 (1997): 149-155.

K. A. Steinmetz, L. H. Kushi, R. M. Bostick, A. R. Folsom, and J. D. Potter, "Vegetables, fruit, and colon cancer in the Iowa women's health study," American Journal of Epidemiology 139, No. 1 (1994): 1-15.

G. Block, B. Patterson, and A. Subar, "Fruit, vegetables, and cancer prevention: a review of the epidemiological evidence," Nutrition and Cancer 18, No. 1 (1992): 1-29.

LEGUMES DECREASE CANCER RISK

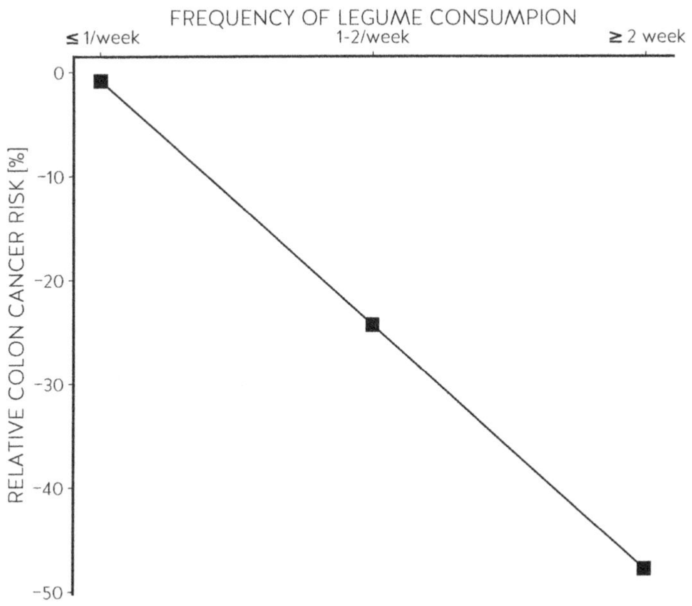

FUN FACT

Legumes are a significant source of protein on plant based diet.

KEY TAKEAWAY

Legumes (for example beans, soy, lentils, and peas) reduce the risk of colon cancer.

- Eating legumes decreases the risk of colon cancer.
- Legumes include beans, peas, and lentils.
- It is not clear if the cancer risk reduction is due to fibers in legumes, or because of some other protective effect. It does not matter - we should eat them anyway.

P. N. Singh and G. E. Fraser, "Dietary risk factors for colon cancer in a low-risk population," American Journal of Epidemiology 148, No. 8 (1998): 761-774.

B. Zhu, Y. Sun, L. Qi, R. Zhong, and X. Miao, "Dietary legume consumption reduces risk of colorectal cancer: evidence from a meta-analysis of cohort studies," Nature: Scientific Reports 5 (2015): 8797.

WHOLE GRAIN AND FIBER DECREASE CANCER RISK

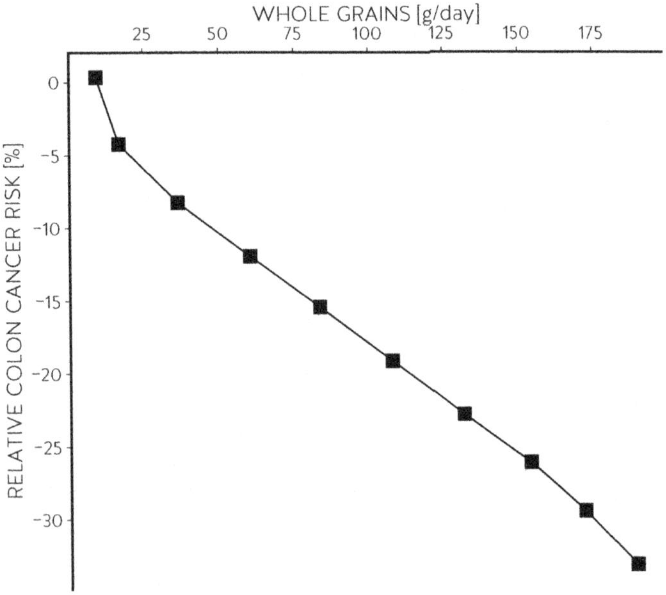

KEY TAKEAWAY

Whole grains (whole grain rye breads, whole grain breads, oatmeal, whole grain cereals, brown rice, and porridge) reduce the risk of colon cancer.

- Dietary fiber and whole grain consumption is associated with linear decreases in the risk of colorectal cancer.
- The cancer risk is reduced by 20% for each three servings of whole grain.

D. Aune, D. S. M. Chan, R. Lau, R. Vieira, D. C. Greenwood, E. Kampman, and T. Norat, "Dietary fibre, whole grains, and risk of colorectal cancer: systematic review and dose-response meta-analysis of prospective studies," BMJ: British Medical Journal 343 (2011): d6617.

VITAMIN D PROTECTS FROM CANCER

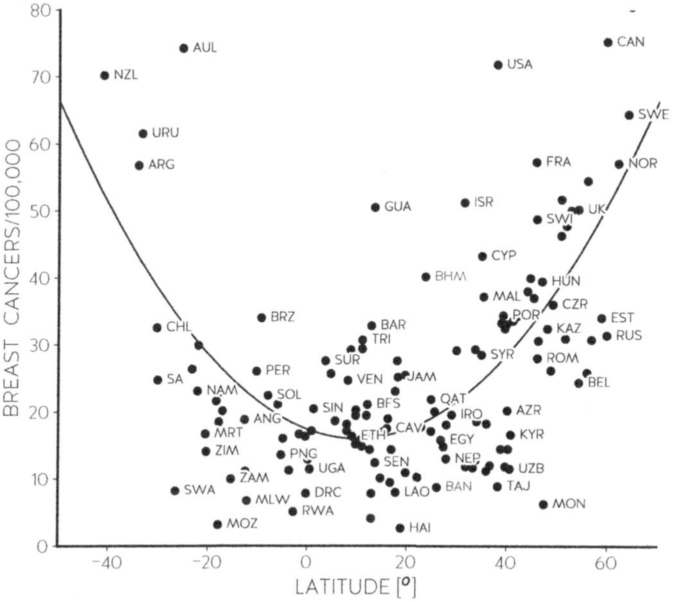

- Cancer incidence rate is lower near the equator where greater solar radiation enables adequate vitamin D levels.
- A clinical trial found that daily supplementation of vitamin D (1000 IU, 25 μg) and calcium reduces the relative cancer risk by 76.8%. Trial size, however, was small and the results need to be confirmed with larger scale trials.
- It is difficult to obtain the optimal amount of vitamin D in modern society from diet and sunlight alone. Vitamin D supplement (1000 IU per day) may reduce cancer risk.

FUN FACT

Vitamin D is fat-soluble. If over consumed, vitamin D can build up to levels that are harmful. The daily maximum dose is 4000 IU and there is no evidence of harm at that level. A blood test can be done to ensure that vitamin D is within the therapeutic range.

KEY TAKEAWAY

Taking vitamin D supplements (1000 IU or 25 μg per day) is smart insurance against cancer.

S. Mohr, C. Garland, E. Gorham, W. Grant, R. Highfill, and F. Garland, "Mapping vitamin D deficiency, breast cancer, and colorectal cancer," In Proceedings of the ESRI International User Conference 1468, Redlands, CA (2005): 1468.

J. M Lappe, D. Travers-Gustafson, K. M. Davies, R. R. Recker, and R. P. Heaney, "Vitamin D and calcium supplementation reduces cancer risk: results of a randomized trial," The American Journal of Clinical Nutrition 85, No. 6 (2007): 1586-1591.

E. D. Gorham et al., "Optimal vitamin D status for colorectal cancer prevention: a quantitative meta analysis," American Journal of Preventive Medicine 32, No. 3 (2007): 210-216.

KEY TAKEAWAYS ON CANCER

An estimated 90-95% of cancers are due to environmental causes. A healthy lifestyle goes a long way toward reducing cancer risks.
Nutritional keys to reduce cancer risks are:

- Avoiding processed meat (salted meats such as bacon and sausage).
- Moderating red meat intake to less than 0.5 lb per week. Red meats include pork, beef, and lamb that are red when raw.
- Evidence about the cancer risk due to white meats (for example chicken) is mixed. It is best to eat these in moderation so the majority of one's diet is from plants that protect from cancers.
- Drinking no more than 1-2 units of alcohol per day.
- Avoiding high glycemic index foods such as sugars, white bread, white rice, breakfast cereals, and white potato.
- Eating more fruit, vegetables, legumes, and whole grains that decrease the cancer risk.
- Daily vitamin D (1000 IU) supplements reduce cancer risk in a clinical trial.

OBESITY & OVERWEIGHT

Obesity is not a sickness but it increases the risk of developing serious diseases including heart disease, diabetes, and cancer. Being overweight also increases strain on joints causing premature wear and tear. For health reasons, it is simply better not to carry too much weight.

The ideal weight/height relationship is commonly quantified by the body mass index (BMI). The BMI is defined as the body mass (in kg) divided by the square of the body height (in meters). Many free online calculators can be found on the web where you can enter your height and weight for an easy calculation of BMI. Commonly accepted BMI ranges are:

- Underweight people: under 18.5 kg/m^2
- Normal weight: 18.5 to 25 kg/m^2
- Overweight: 25 to 30 kg/m^2
- Obese: over 30 kg/m^2

This chapter covers how dietary choices affect BMI and how BMI affects the quality of life and life expectancy.

The desire to lose weight is quite common but the reality is that the majority of people gain weight year after year in steady progression. Common weight loss diets work in the short term but long-term success rates are dismal. A lasting change requires nothing less than a lifestyle change. Hence, our focus is on developing eating patterns with long-term success in achieving and maintaining normal BMI.

HIGH BMI REDUCES LIFE EXPECTANCY

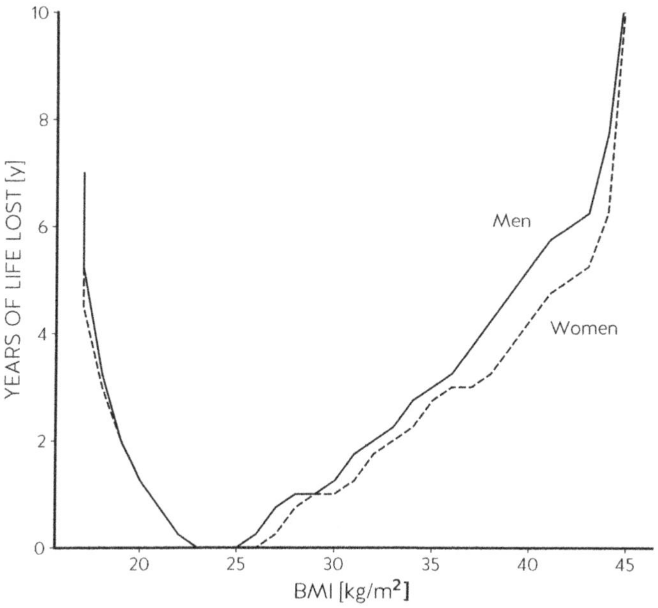

FUN FACT
More than 70% of Americans are overweight ore obese.

KEY TAKEAWAY
Normal BMI maximizes life expectancy.

- High body mass index (BMI) is a risk factor for heart disease, diabetes, and cancer, which shorten one's lifespan.
- BMI=25 kg/m^2 is the cutoff point for normal weight because BMI > 25 kg/m^2 lowers the life expectancy.
- Being underweight (BMI <18.5kg/m^2) is also associated with lower life expectancy; however, low BMI may be the result of a fatal illness, such as cancer, and not the underlying cause of low life expectancy. There is no evidence that healthy non-smokers that are underweight have lower life expectancy.

K. R. Fontaine, D. T. Redden, C. Wang, A. O. Westfall, D. B. Allison, "Years of life lost due to obesity," Journal of American Medical Association 289, No. 2 (2003): 187-193.

INCREASE IN BMI AFFECTS HEALTH NEGATIVELY EVEN IN THE NORMAL RANGE

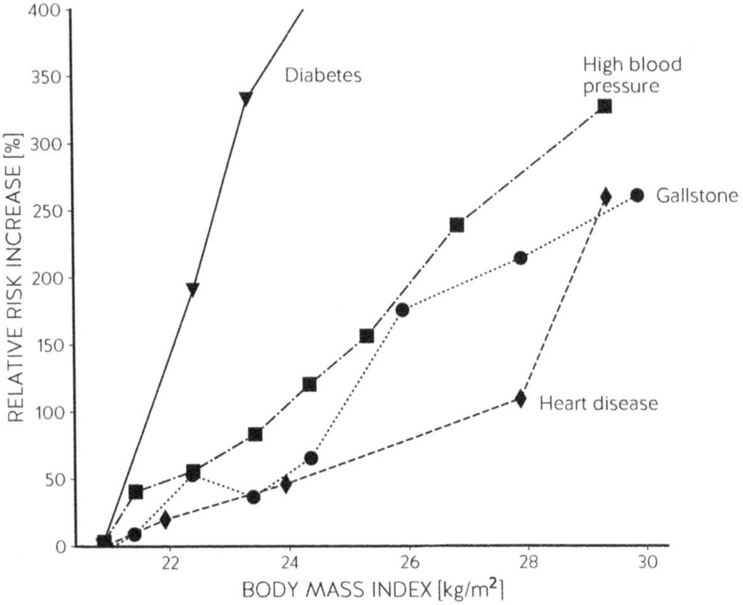

- Increase in BMI increases disease risks even at the normal levels (BMI range of 20 to 25 kg/m^2).
- Diabetes risk is especially sensitive to body mass. The risk of diabetes increases by more than 400% with a BMI change from 21 to 25 kg/m^2.

W. Willett, Eat, drink, and be healthy: the Harvard Medical School guide to healthy eating, Simon and Schuster, 2017.

FUN FACT

There is no reason for BMI to increase during the adult life. If your BMI has risen since you were 20 years old, you could benefit from lowering your body weight.

KEY TAKEAWAY

Higher BMI means increased disease risks even in the normal BMI range of 20 to 25 kg/m^2. Ideally, the BMI should be in the lower end of the normal BMI range.

BMI AND CHOLESTEROL LEVELS ARE LINKED

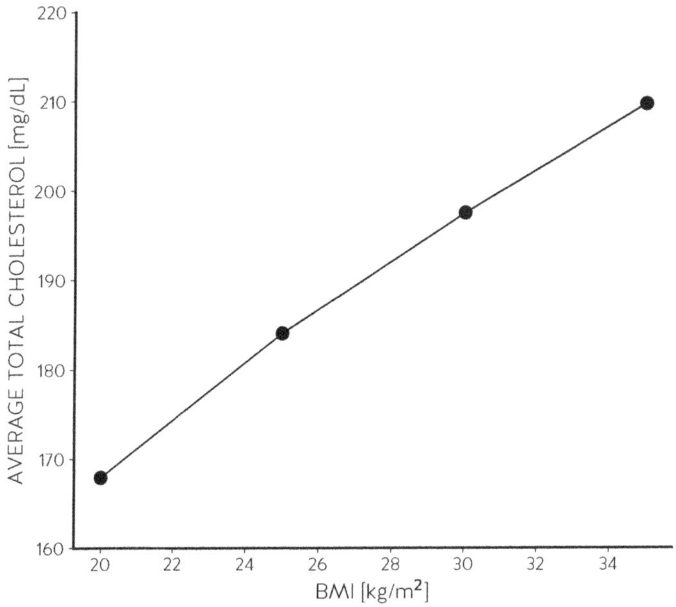

KEY TAKEAWAY
If you stay on a healthy diet and your body mass drops, you should see corresponding long-term improvement in cholesterol levels.

- Cholesterol levels correlate with BMI. Lowering BMI by just 1 kg/m^2 is associated with 3 mg/dL lower total cholesterol level.
- In addition to total cholesterol, LDL cholesterol is also reduced and HDL cholesterol is slightly improved.
- While cholesterol levels can respond quickly to changes in diet, body-weight changes are slower. After changing a diet, we can, therefore, expect a fast initial change in cholesterol followed by a more gradual change as body weight is reduced.

F. Abbasi, B. W. Brown, C. Lamendola, T. McLaughlin, and G. M. Reaven, "Relationship between obesity, insulin resistance, and coronary heart disease risk," Journal of the American College of Cardiology 40, No. 5 (2002): 937-943.

Y.-H. Hsu, S. A. Venners, H. A. Terwedow, Y. Feng, T. Niu, Z. Li, N. Laird, J. D Brain, S. R. Cummings, M. L. Bouxsein, C. J. Rosen, and X. Xu, "Relation of body composition, fat mass, and serum lipids to osteoporotic fractures and bone mineral density in Chinese men and women," The American Journal of Clinical Nutrition 83, No. 1 (2006): 146-154.

WEIGHT LOSS DIETS WORK ... INITIALLY

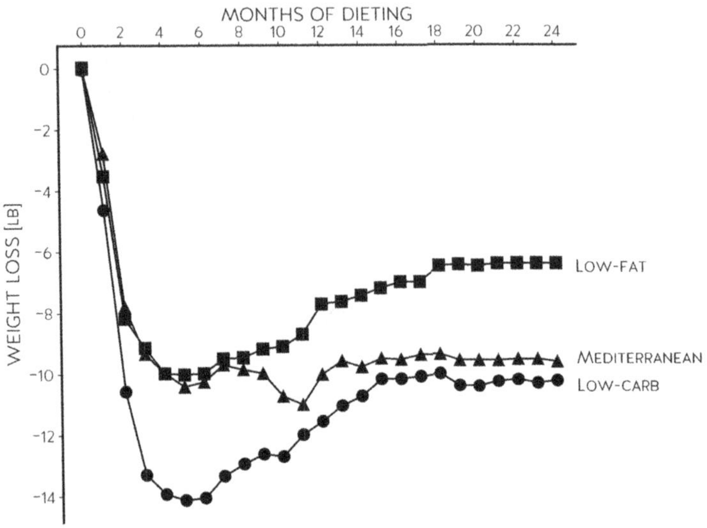

FUN FACT
Diet studies typically last 6 months or less. Very few studies last more than 1 year. This time span is too short to measure long-term effects.

KEY TAKEAWAY
Most diets can result in a quick weight drop, but long term weight reduction is more difficult.

- Most weight loss diets result in initial weight loss; however, after 6 months, one's weight typically stabilizes or even bounces back.
- There is no magical diet that results in fast weight loss, month after month.
- Successful, long-term weight loss is the reverse of weight gain: slow and steady progress. Years of weight gain will likely take years to fully reverse.

I. Shai, D. Schwarzfuchs, Y. Henkin, D. R. Shahar, S. Witkow, I. Greenberg, R. Golan, D. Fraser, A. Bolotin, H. Vardi, O. Tangi-Rozental, R. Zuk-Ramot, B. Sarusi, D. Brickner, Z. Schwartz, E. Sheiner, R. Marko, E. Katorza, J. Thiery, G. Martin Fiedler, M. Bluher, M. Stumvoll, and M. J. Stampfer, "Weight loss with a low-carbohydrate, Mediterranean, or low-fat diet," New England Journal of Medicine 359, No. 3 (2008): 229-241.

ALTERNATE-DAY FASTING LOWERS WEIGHT

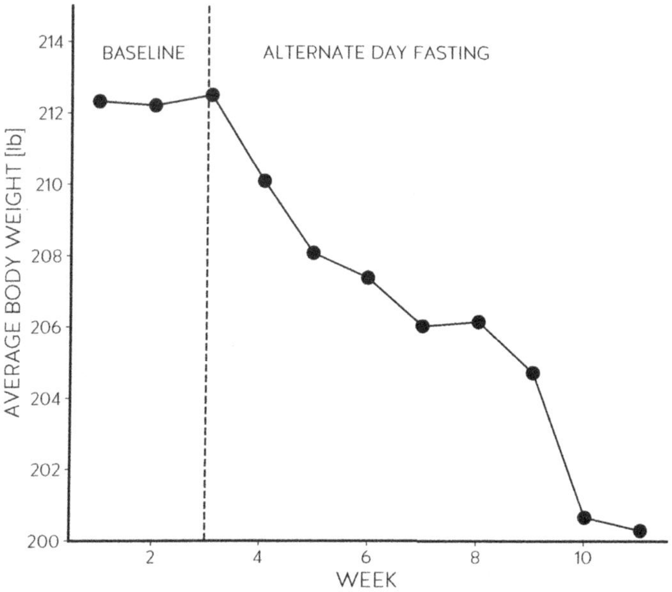

FUN FACT
Although fasting is trendy, the results after one year of fasting do not differ much compared to daily calorie reduction. You can experiment with both approaches and choose the one that is easier to follow.

- In alternate-day fasting, the energy intake is reduced to less than 500 kcal on every other day. On non-fasting days, energy consumption is kept normal.
- Alternate-day fasting results in fast weight reduction in an obese person.
- Importantly, muscle mass is not lost in alternate-day fasting. The weight loss is due to fat loss. This is an advantage over continuous calorie restriction that typically results in both fat and muscle mass loss.
- Alternate-day fasting also lowers total cholesterol (p. 55) and improves insulin sensitivity.
- Although the alternate-day protocol is the most studied fasting protocol, other types of fasts may be easier to implement and stick to. Fasting just two nonconsecutive days a week is a popular option.

- Fasting is very effective because it reduces calorie intake and lowers insulin levels (p. 83) thus encouraging the body to burn fat.
- By all indications, sustained alternate-day fasting helps maintain normal body weight without a loss in muscle mass.

K. A. Varady, S. Bhutani, E. C. Church, and M. C. Klempel, "Short-term modified alternate-day fasting: a novel dietary strategy for weight loss and cardioprotection in obese adults," The American Journal of Clinical Nutrition 90, No. 9 (2009): 1138-1143.

M. C. Klempel, C. M. Kroeger, and K. A. Varady, "Alternate day fasting (ADF) with a high-fat diet produces similar weight loss and cardio-protection as ADF with a low-fat diet," Metabolism 62, No. 1 (2013): 137-143.

J. F. Trepanowski, C. M. Kroeger, A. Barnosky, M. C. Klempel, S. Bhutani, K. K. Hoddy, K. Gabel, S. Freels, J. Rigdon, J. Rood, E. Ravussin, K. A. Varady, "Effect of alternate-day fasting on weight loss, weight maintenance, and cardioprotection among metabolically healthy obese adults: a randomized clinical trial," JAMA Internal Medicine 177, No. 7 (2017): 930-938.

KEY TAKEAWAY

Alternate-day fasting can be an effective way to lower weight quickly. An advantage of alternate-day fasting is that it is relatively simple to implement, but it does require tolerating the feeling of hunger on fast days.

WHOLE FOODS HAVE HIGH SATIETY

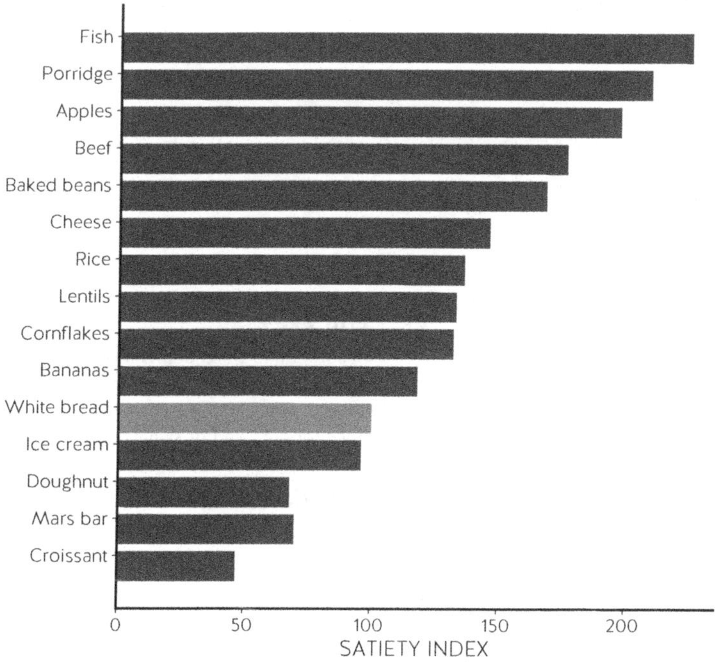

FUN FACT

In clinical trials, people tend to eat significantly higher amount calories when served processed foods than when eating whole foods.

KEY TAKEAWAY

Eating whole foods is a naturally slimming diet. Eating processed foods is a naturally fattening diet.

- Satiety index measures how filling a food is per calorie. To feel full, you need to eat larger calorie amounts of foods with a low satiety index than high satiety index foods.
- Calorie dense baked foods such as cake, croissants, doughnuts, and white bread have a low satiety index.
- Ultraprocessed foods in general tend to be very energy dense and have low satiety index.
- Simple whole foods such as fruit, fish, meat, whole grains tend to have high satiety index.

S. Holt, J. C. Brand Miller, P. Petocz, and E. Farmakalidis, "A satiety index of common foods," European journal of clinical nutrition 49, No. 9 (1995): 675-690.

SLEEP DEPRIVATION CAUSES OVEREATING

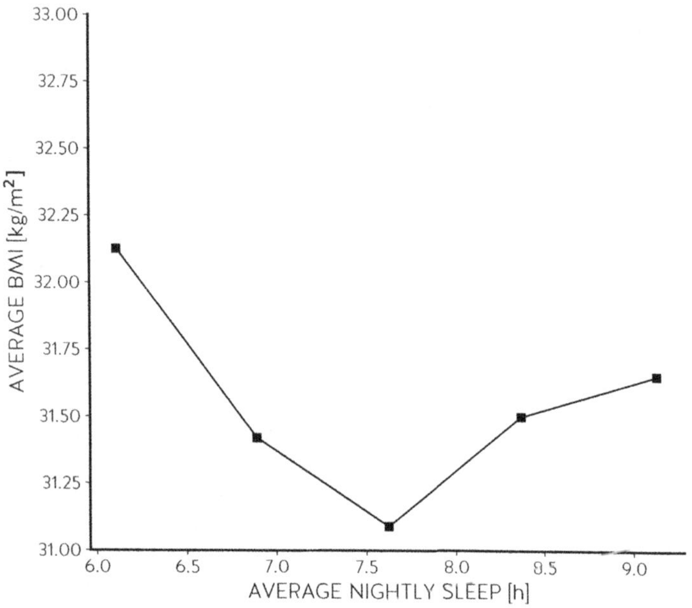

FUN FACT

In addition to sleep deprivation, stress in general can cause over eating ("stress eating") and prefer-ence for fatty and/or sweet food.

KEY TAKEAWAY

Try to get enough sleep to be well rested.

- Short sleep duration of less than 7 hours per day is associated with higher average BMI.
- In clinical studies, sleep deprivation causes increased hunger and significant increase in calorie intake.
- Long sleep also associated with higher average body weight; however, this association is likely due to an underlying illness such as depression. There is no evidence that being too well rested increases body weight.

OS. Taheri, L. Lin, D. Austin, T. Young, and E. Mignot, "Short sleep duration is associated with reduced leptin, elevated ghrelin, and increased body mass index," PLOS Medicine 1, No. 3 (2004): e62.

M.-P. St-Onge, A. McReynolds, Z. B. Trivedi, A. L. Roberts, M. Sy, and J. Hirsch, "Sleep restriction leads to increased activation of brain regions sensitive to food stimuli,"The American Journal of Clinical Nutrition 95, No. 4 (2012): 818-824.

S. Guyenet, The Hungry Brain: Outsmarting the Instincts that Make Us Overeat, Macmillan, 2017.

BMI IS CONSISTENTLY NORMAL ON A PLANT-BASED DIET

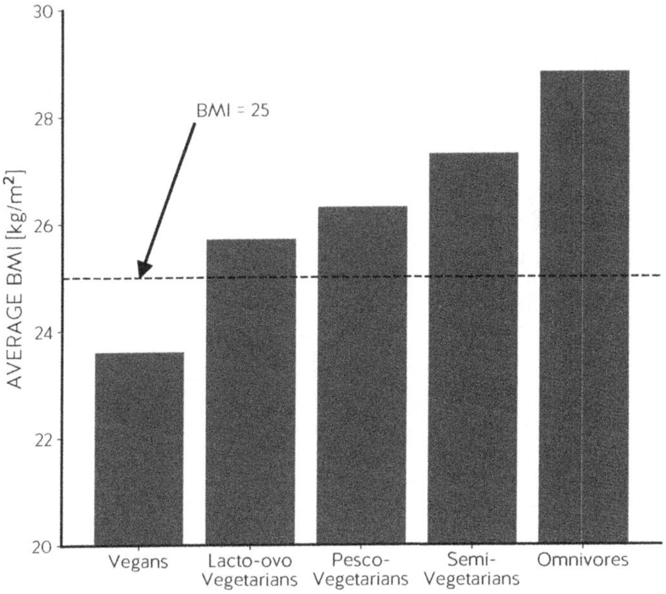

KEY TAKEAWAY
A plant-based diet consistently achieves normal BMI.

- A vegan diet that includes only plants (all fruits, vegetables, legumes (dried beans and peas), grains, seeds and nuts) is associated with a normal average body mass index (BMI).
- All other diets result in, on average, higher than normal BMI. The BMI correlates with amount of animal products in diet:

    Lacto-ovo vegetarian diet includes dairy and eggs.

    Pesco-vegetarian diet also includes fish.

    Semi-vegetarians eat meat just once per week.

    Omnivores can eat all animal products and have the highest average BMI.

- Attaining a normal BMI is possible through these diets but may require a conscious effort to exercise and to control calorie intake.

S. G. De Biase, S. F. C. Fernandes, R. J. Gianini, and J. L. Duarte, "Vegetarian diet and cholesterol and triglycerides levels," Arquivos Brasileiros de Cardiologia 88, No. 1 (2007): 35-39.

KEY TAKEAWAYS ON BMI

A normal BMI is desirable for health and longevity reasons. Ideally, the BMI should be in the lower end of the normal range of 20 to 25 kg/m^2 to minimize disease risks.

Unfortunately, we have not discovered the miracle diet that results in a perfect body with no effort. Most dieting efforts result in an initial drop in body weight but the fast weight decrease is usually not sustained and weight may actually come back. Recognizing the challenge and setting the right expectation is the first step toward tackling this problem.

Weight gain is typically a gradual process. Average Americans gain 1-2 lb of weight every year which builds up over decades. Reversing this weight gain can take years which is not addressed in shorter term weight loss studies. The best chance to attain a normal body weight may be to adopt an evidence-based diet pattern that results in a low BMI.

Whole foods such as fruits, beans, whole grains, meat, and fish tend to have high satiety. In contrast, processed foods have low satiety and one tends to over eat them before feeling full.

Lack of sufficient sleep can lead to eating too much. Try to sleep enough to be well rested.

People following a vegan diet commonly achieve normal BMI. In fact, the vegan diet is the only diet that consistently achieves a BMI < 25 kg/m^2 in Western societies. Following other diets may require a more conscious effort to manage body weight. Fasting is one effective option to control body weight.

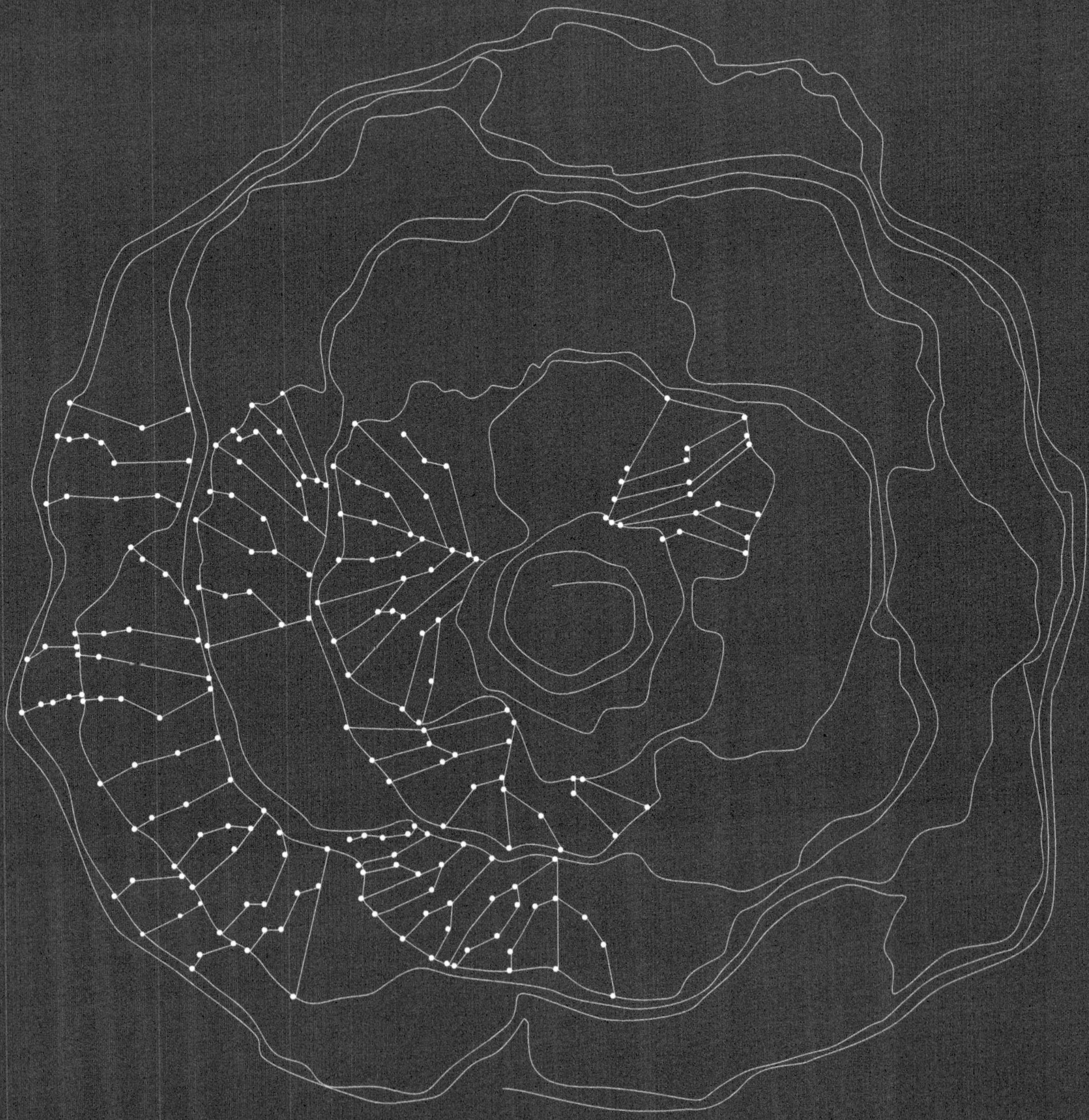

PART II

INTERPRETATION

The remainder of the book puts the research into action. Everyone eats differently and it would be foolish to claim that there is one diet that fits everyone. However, it is also true that everyone can improve their dietary health. If you prefer a certain diet, whether it is Paleo, vegan, or something more standard, I'll show you how you can improve it by making a few tweaks.

First, I will offer a set of measurable targets to improve your dietary health. These targets allow you to quantify how close you are to optimal health. Next, I will cover the dietary "means" for reaching these targets. It is up to you to choose which means you adopt. Feel free to experiment to find what works for you.

TARGETS

The approach taken here is different than other nutritional books. The standard "best-seller" formula is to promise health and longevity by following certain dietary guidelines. Here we'll take the reverse approach: We set measurable goals and offer dietary guidelines or "means" to reach those goals. It is up to you to choose the dietary "means" that work for you. The nutrition is not the end goal. Staying healthy is the primary target.

I am assuming that you want to live as long as possible with the best possible health. This means stopping 1.) the development of heart disease, 2.) avoiding type-2 diabetes, 3.) maintaining ideal body weight, and 4.) reducing the cancer probability to the lowest possible risk level. The first three targets are measurable:

- *Heart disease*

  Heart disease risk can be quantified by a cholesterol measurement. Everyone should know their cholesterol numbers. Evidence from large scale studies covering thousands of people across many cultures shows that total cholesterol less than 150 mg/dL (3.9 mmol/L) minimizes the risk of heart disease (p. 18). Indigenous People who are free of heart disease have cholesterol levels less than 150 mg/dL (p. 27) and there is no reason we should be less healthy. Unlike Indigenous People who must eat the food locally available and in season, we have the privilege of benefiting from extensive research and easy access to an abundance of healthy food choices.

  The optimal LDL level is less than 70 mg/dL (1.8 mmol/L). There is no evidence that LDL can be too low for heart health (p. 19).

  The interpretation of HDL is more complicated. Low HDL (defined as <50 mg/dL or <1.3 mmol/L in women and <40 mg/dL or 1.0 mmol/L in men) increases risk of cardiovascular disease especially in combination with high LDL. Higher levels of HDL, however, may not offer additional protection and widespread practice of calculating the ratio of LDL to HDL may not be useful[20]. HDL can be increased by eating more fat and exercising (which is a more desirable approach), however, our primary focus is on LDL and total cholesterol as these are directly linked to heart disease risk.

Comparison of ideal cholesterol and generally recommended "normal" values is shown in Table 1 below. As you can see, there is a fairly big gap between the ideal values and "standard guideline" values. Here is the catch: The normal values are a compromise between what is generally thought to be both achievable by the average population and what results in an acceptable risk. The target of <200 mg/dL is achievable by relatively small improvements to the Standard Ameracan diet but it is not enough to stop the progression of cardiovascular disease. Changing the official target to 150 mg/dL, however, would mean that >98% of Americans would fail to meet the recommendation, which understandably is holding back the health authorities. Nevertheless, the medical authorities are slowly moving towards lower targets: LDL cholesterol target was lowered from <130 mg/dL to <100 mg/dL in 2004 and <70 mg/dL is already recommended to anyone with a "high risk" of heart disease.

TABLE 1. COMPARISON OF CHOLESTEROL GUIDELINES

	GENERAL GUIDELINES	OPTIMAL LEVELS
Total Cholesterol	<200 mg/dL (5.2 mmol/L)	<150 mg/dL (3.9 mmol/L)
LDL	<100 mg/dL (2.6 mmol/L)	<70 mg/dL (1.8 mmol/L)
HDL	>40 mg/dL (1.0 mmol/L) for men >50 mg/dL (1.3 mmol/L) for women	

Cholesterol is part of the lipid panel test that is typically measured every few years but it can be measured more often, for example every six months, to see how the cholesterol levels are affected by diet changes. The test can be ordered by your doctor, in which case it is probably covered for those with the Affordable Care Act. The test can also be ordered online without visiting a doctor. This approach is especially attractive if you want to test your cholesterol more often than is covered by your insurance. A typical cost for the lipid panel is around $30-$50. Remember to fast for 12 hours before the test.

In addition to cholesterol levels, it may be prudent to check the homocysteine level, as it is an independent risk factor for coronary heart disease (p. 43). Many people, and especially vegans, have an inadequate B12-vitamin intake, which can lead to dangerously high homocysteine level. The homocysteine level should be less than 12 μmole/L (ideally <10 μmole/L).

Normal blood pressure is defined as less than 120 mmHg (systolic) / 80 mmHg (diastolic) but measurable complications of high blood pressure begin to appear already at 115 mmHg (systolic). It is typical that blood pressure increases with age; however, this is not normal but may be a sign of hardening of the arteries due to an unhealthy diet. In cultures with low prevalence of heart disease, the blood pressure stays normal through life.

- *Diabetes risk*

  A simple fasting glucose measurement quantifies type-2 diabetes risk (p. 69). Fasting glucose should be less than 100 mg/dL (ideally less than 80 mg/dL). Fasting glucose is commonly measured as part of the lipid panel.

  Another easy lab test is hemoglobin A1c, which measures average blood glucose level. The normal range for the hemoglobin A1c level is between 4% and 5.6% but values higher than 5% mark progressively increased diabetes risk (p. 70).

- *Normal body mass index*

  The normal body mass index (BMI) ranges from 20 to 25 kg/m^2. Maintaining BMI in the lower end of this range reduces the risk of heart disease, type-2 diabetes (p. 69 and 102), and cancer (p. 91).

  Body mass index (BMI) is calculated by the following formula: mass/(height*height) where mass is in kg and height is in meters. For example, a 1.75 m tall person weighing 67 kg has a BMI of 21.9 (67/(1.75*1.75) = 21.9). If calculations and international units are not your thing, there are many free online BMI calculators where you can enter your weight and height in any units.

- *Minimal cancer risk*

  Unfortunately, there is no easy measurement for our fourth target of minimizing the cancer risk; however, by following the nutritional guidelines outlined here, one can reduce cancer risk by at least 30% (p. 87)[13]. The guidelines for avoiding cancer are largely the same as those given for avoiding heart disease and diabetes. In addition, to reduce cancer risk, I do recommend avoiding processed meat products and excess alcohol.

MEANS

The targets are clear: we want to avoid heart disease and type-2 diabetes with near certainty, have normal BMI, and reduce cancer risk as much as possible. The science to achieve these targets is also clear: Eating a mostly plant-based, low-glycemic-index diet is the default starting point for any healthy diet. This might appear to be too good to be true but by eating vegetables and avoiding high glycemic index foods, we can avoid the most common health problems. The same diet works to minimize heart disease, diabetes, and cancer risk!

Vegetarian diets and especially the vegan diet are associated with lower BMI values, lower prevalence of higher blood pressure, lower prevalence of the metabolic syndrome, diabetes, and heart disease. These positive outcomes are observed in large scale population studies even though vegetarians are commonly deficient in vitamin B12 (particularly vegans), iron, calcium, zinc, and vitamin D. What could we achieve with a plant-based diet that has the sufficient amount of these nutrients? This has not been studied but a diet like this is probably the best option for optimal health.

The advice to eat a plant-based diet is not controversial. Everyone agrees that vegetables are healthy and we should eat more of them. In fact, in population studies, the vegan diet is associated with the lowest average cholesterol levels and adding even small amounts of animal products to the diet increases cholesterol levels.

Eating a pure vegan diet, however, is not the only way to minimize heart disease risk. Many Indigenous Cultures consume animal products but are by and large free of heart disease and diabetes. It may be impossible to revert to a hunter-gatherer lifestyle in modern settings, but we can adopt aspects of a hunter-gatherer lifestyle to maintain optimal health. This includes avoidance of processed foods, avoiding industrial vegetable oils, exercising daily, fasting periodically, ensuring sufficient vitamin B and D intake, and obtaining the right balance of Omega-3 and 6 fats. The more one deviates from a pure plant-based diet, the more important these aspects from the Indigenous Cultures become.

The Evidence Based Diet has three elements: don'ts, moderates and do's. Don'ts are the things to avoid or eat with extreme moderation as they are harmful. Moderates are things that are not harmful and may even be beneficial in moderation. Moderates are safe to eat a few times a week. Do's are beneficial and there is no limit to their consumption. Since do's are the cornerstone of the healthy diet, one should not veer into moderates unless the daily quota of do's is getting filled.

DON'TS

As is evidenced by the growing obesity epidemic, we eat too much and consume too many calories. We should, however, eat even more fruits and vegetables. To solve this dilemma, we should eliminate or significantly reduce the intake of some foods.

Don'ts are foods that are high in calories but low in nutritional value. These are the foods one should avoid or eat very sparingly:

- *Refined carbohydrates*

  These include sugary drinks and snacks, white bread, pasta, and white rice. They are calorically dense, have a high glycemic index, and contain almost no nutritional value. Consuming these leads to insulin spikes that may cause insulin resistance, obesity, and type-2 diabetes (p. 71). A diet with a high glycemic index also increases the risk of heart disease (p. 30) and cancer (p. 92). Talk about a lose-lose!

  In addition, sugary snacks are surprisingly addictive. In brains scan studies, high glycemic index meals are shown to stimulate brain regions associated with reward in a manner similar to drugs[4]. High glycemic index meals also lead to an increased sensation of hunger after the meal and can change the taste palate so that healthy foods won't seem as tasty. It is much easier to avoid sugar snacks completely than to moderate their consumption.

- *Processed meats*

  Processed meat consumption, including bacon, sausage, and salami, increases cancer risks. The evidence is so strong that the World Health Organization (WHO) now lists processed meats as Type 1 carcinogen.

- *Industrial vegetable oils*

  Vegetable oils, including canola oil, corn oil, and cottonseed oil are high in Omega-6 fats and contain almost no Omega-3 fats. High use of processed vegetables oils makes it impossible to maintain a healthy Omega-6 to Omega-3 ratio that is important for heart health (p. 41). Instead, I recommend using olive oil. For meals where the taste of olive oil is not acceptable, avocado oil and nut oils are good alternatives.

- *Oils high in saturated and trans fats*

  Saturated fats raise LDL cholesterol levels (p. 38). Avoid cooking with animal-based fats (for example lard and butter) that contain both saturated fats and trans fats. Among vegetable oils, palm oil and coconut oil are also high in saturated fat.

MODERATES

These foods are good in moderation as long as the cholesterol levels are in the optimal range:

- *Red meat*

  Red meat is linked to colon cancer (p. 88) and cardiovascular disease (p. 48). Limit to 0.5 lb (250 g) per week to minimize cancer and heart disease risk. If your cholesterol does not reach the target levels, consider eliminating red meat completely from your diet.

- *Other animal products*

  Animal products including chicken and dairy products are a good source of protein; however, even relatively low amounts can raise your cholesterol levels (p. 25). It is not possible to provide consumption limit recommendations for these foods due to a lack of research. My advice is to consume these foods only a few days per week so that your diet is primarily comprised of the really good stuff (plants). Having meatless days also helps in discovering new ways to cook and eat, which will be a key in permanently shifting your diet toward a more plant-based mixture of foods. If your cholesterol levels stay too high, reduce the consumption of animal products even further.

- *Fish*

  Fish contain healthy Omega-3s in long chain form (EPA and DHA) that is not available in plants. Unfortunately, large fish are often contaminated with mercury, PCB, and dioxin. Also, consuming a large amount of fish can raise cholesterol levels. My best advice is to occasionally eat small fish such as sardines. Vegans can obtain EPA and DHA from algae derived supplements. I do not recommend eating fish oil supplements as they raise LDL cholesterol levels.

- *Starchy vegetables*

  Starchy vegetables such as white potatoes and corn have low nutritional value and can cause a disproportionately large insulin response. Moderation is acceptable. Eat with vinegar to reduce blood glucose response (p. 81).

- *Alcohol*

  Alcohol may be beneficial to heart health in small quantities but increases cancer risk in larger quantities (p. 90). Limit to 1-2 units per day.

DO'S

The do's, the good stuff, include all the food that keeps the body working at optimal health:

- *Green leafy vegetables*

  Green leafy vegetables are the healthiest foods on the planet and are easy to recognize at the grocery store. I recommend stocking up on collard greens, kale, turnip greens, swiss chard, bok choy, mustard greens, spinach, and different lettuces. Eat them in salads, in green smoothies, steam them or add them in soups. Humans have gathered and eaten these greens for thousands of years and they are the true Paleo diet food. Make sure you eat them daily to reduce risk of hearth disease (p. 32), diabetes (p. 77), and cancer (p. 93).

- *Other non-starchy vegetables*

  Non-starchy vegetables include asparagus, squash, zucchini, carrots, broccoli, cucumber, peppers,onions, and tomatoes. You want to eat these daily.

- *Legumes*

  Legumes including beans, peas, soy, and lentils contain plant protein, which makes them very important for vegan diets. Legumes are also linked to lower cancer (p. 95) and heart disease risk.

- *Sweet potatoes*

  Unlike white potatoes, sweet potatoes do not cause a large spike in insulin levels.

- *Whole grains*

  Whole grains are slow to digest and have a low glycemic index. Studies link whole grains to reduced risk of diabetes, cancer (p. 96), and heart disease (p. 34). Eating oats may be especially helpful as they can significantly lower cholesterol levels (p. 33).

- *Berries*

  Berries reduce diabetes risk (p. 75). They also contain a large amount antioxidants and fiber. And they lower cholesterol[5]. Eat them daily.

- *Nuts*

  In populations studies, nuts are associated with a 50% reduction of heart disease when eaten daily (p. 47). This is nothing less than a miracle; however, nuts are calorically dense foods and easy to overeat. Don't eat more than a closed handful a day (about 1/4 cup). Walnuts are especially healthy as they contain Omega-3s.

- *Mushrooms*

  Mushrooms are another great addition to any diet. They're low in calories and are great sources of fiber and protein. They also provide many important nutrients including selenium and potassium.

- *Omega-3 fatty acids*

  Omega-6/Omega-3 ratio may be crucial for vascular health (p. 41). Omega-3s come in three main forms: short chain ALA, long chain EPA, and DHA. Evidence from heart disease prevention studies suggests that daily intakes of between 1.5 grams and 3.0 grams of ALA Omega-3 fatty acids are very beneficial.

  Two tablespoons of ground flaxseed provides about 1.6 grams of ALA. You can add them in smoothies, salads, or on top of other foods. Flaxseeds need to be ground or they cannot be digested. Alternatively, 1/4 cup of walnuts contains 2.5 grams of ALA. Eating walnuts daily covers the ALA needs with ease.

Long chain Omega-3s (EPA and DHA) are not readily available in plants. The human body can convert short chain ALA into EPA and DHA but this conversion mechanism is disrupted if one eats food rich in Omega-6 fatty acids, which block the conversion path. Therefore, it is important to avoid industrially processed vegetable oils that are high in Omega-6 fatty acids (one of the don'ts!).

The conversion mechanism may also become impaired as we get older. It may be prudent to also obtain some long chain Omega-3s by consuming some fish or EPA and DHA containing supplements.

- *Vitamin B12*

  Vitamin B12 plays a key role in the normal functioning of the brain and nervous system. Together with foliates derived from plants, especially green leafy vegetables, B12 is important in controlling our homocysteine level. Strong evidence gathered over the past decade suggests that even slightly elevated homocysteine levels increase our risk of heart disease and stroke.

  Vitamin B12 is produced by bacteria. It is found in animal products but not in vegetables. Vegans must consume B12 fortified foods or take supplements to avoid B-12 deficiency. B12 supplementation is also recommended for meat eaters as they do not usually reach optimal B12 levels either (p. 44).

  The following dosage maximizes the B12 blood levels:

  > Eat fortified foods three or four times a day to get at least three micrograms (mcg or μg) of B12 a day or
  >
  > Take one B12 supplement daily providing at least 250 micrograms or
  >
  > Take a weekly B12 supplement providing at least 2500 micrograms.

  Eating more than the above offers no benefit as the excess B12 is excreted in urine.

- *Vitamin D*

  There is growing evidence linking vitamin D deficiency to heart attacks (p. 56) and cancers (p. 97) . In modern society, we do not typically get enough sunlight to produce optimal levels of vitamin D. Current evidence supports eating 1,000 IU of vitamin D daily (1,000 IU equals 25 μg). D-vitamin is not water soluble and it is possible to eat too much of it. The maximum daily dosage is 4,000 IU and there is no evidence of harm at that level.

- *Apple cider vinegar*
  Eating apple cider vinegar with starchy foods helps to moderate blood glucose and insulin levels (p. 81). Apple cider vinegar may also help in lowering cholesterol levels (p. 53). Consume one or two tablespoons per day, for example, in salads.

- *Water*
  Drinking 5 cups of water per day minimizes the death risk (p. 57).

- *Sleep*
  Remember to sleep until you are well rested. We sleep more than 1/3 of our life because it is important (p. 108). If sleeping were optional, millions of years of evolution would have eliminated it. It hasn't.

- *Fast*
  Fasting 1 to 3 times per week is optional but it's an effective way to lower body mass (p. 105) and cholesterol levels (p. 55). More on this in the next section.

I want to stress the importance of eating the do's in quantities. An apple a day does not do much but eating eight servings of fruits and vegetables every day does marvels to reduce cancer and heart disease risk. Moreover, the benefits from different do's do add up. For example, oat bran, greens, and nuts each result in a small improvement in cholesterol but combined they can reduce cholesterol by 30%[14]. I urge you to make the best use of all tools available for reaching your optimal health.

FASTING

The two options to reduce calorie intake are either to 1.) eat smaller amounts at meal time or 2.) eat fewer meals. In other words, we can either eat less or less frequently. It turns out that many people find eating less frequently to be the easier solution compared to eating less.

Skipping meals or fasting is an often overlooked element of many healthy diets. The highly praised Mediterranean diet incorporates fasting. In fact, the Greek Orthodox fast two days per week and include longer fasts throughout the year. Hunter-gatherers, who do not have easy access to packaged foods, periodically fast by necessity (unsuccessful hunt) or choice (relaxing is more appealing than gathering food, gathering firewood, making a fire, and cooking)[6].

In clinical trials, periodic fasting for 24 hours effectively lowers body fat and total cholesterol levels without a loss in muscle mass. The lack of muscle loss is the major advantage of fasting in comparison to continuous energy restriction. Typical weight loss diet regimes that continuously reduce the calorie intake result in both fat and muscle loss, which is undesirable.

Most studies have focused on the alternate-day fasting (ADF) protocol where an eating day is followed by a fasting day. This might be difficult to follow long term. An easier approach involves fasting two nonconsecutive days per week (5/2 fasting or intermittent fasting). There are fewer studies on intermittent fasting but the available evidence suggests that fasting may be more beneficial than continuous energy restriction[7].

The rationale for fasting is easy to understand: After a meal, the human body is in a fed state that lasts 3-4 hours. In the fed state, energy is stored in human cells, the insulin levels are high, and LDL cholesterol levels are elevated[8]. If you eat every few hours, you are constantly in a fed state. Fasting breaks this cycle allowing the body to rest and use stored energy reserves. Evolution has prepared the human body to cope remarkably well with periods of scarcity and growing evidence suggests that the human body not only survives but thrives from fasting.

The most common approaches to the intermittent fasting are 1) *calorie restriction* for 24 hours, 2) *total fast* for 24 hours, and 3) daily *time restricted eating*. The *calorie restriction* approach limits total calorie intake to 500 kcal on fasting days, which is less than 1/4 of typical daily calorie intake. The best foods during fasting days are vegetables such as carrots, broccoli, asparagus, lettuce or peas that contain a lot of fiber. These high-fiber foods both fill the stomach and are low in calories. Other good options include avocados and nuts. They are more energy dense foods but do not elevate the insulin levels as much, so you may feel less hungry in the hours following the snack.

The *total fast* approach allows only non-caloric drinks such as water and small amounts of coffee or tea. Some find the total fast to be easier to implement as it does not involve calorie counting.

Time-restricted eating is yet another popular option for fasting where eating is restricted to a six hour window; for example, between 12 and 6 pm. This allows for eating lunch and dinner while fasting for 18 hours daily. My suggestion is to try different approaches and see what works for you.

A common misconception about fasting is that one just eats more on non-fast days. This may happen, but not enough to compensate for the reduction in calories during the fast. Somehow humans naturally reduce the total energy intake when eating fewer meals.

Many are intimidated by the idea of fasting. Most Westerners have never experienced more than an overnight fast (from evening to sunrise) and the idea of not eating during the daytime may sound strange or even frightening. However, fasting is practiced widely outside the Western world by nearly one third of the world's population for mostly religious reasons. Muslims fast. Buddhists fast. The Greek Orthodox fast.

If you are new to fasting, it may be a good idea to start small and just skip one meal, for example a breakfast or a lunch. The first time may feel difficult but fasting becomes easier with practice. Once you are comfortable skipping one meal, try skipping two. Then try a whole day without eating or eating less than 500 kcal.

A major benefit of fasting is that it can change one's relationship to food and eating. I can speak from personal experience. My days used to be planned around eating certain hours whether or not I was hungry. And if I did not eat at the meal times, I would get irritable. The first time I skipped breakfast, I felt horrible but I found that my body adapted to fasting with practice. Now I have the freedom to eat only when I choose to. And when I do eat, the food tastes better as I usually have waited until I am truly hungry.

An added benefit of fasting is that it solves a major problem encountered with any non-standard diet: what to do in social occasions such as cocktail parties if there is no healthy food available? Instead of eating the available unhealthy food, fasting offers a fabulous third option: to relax and feel slightly smuggish observing others gorging on unhealthy foods. (For an ultimate smug trip, visit a fast food restaurant, order unsweetened tea or coffee, and enjoy the better-than-others sensation).

Important notes:

- Don't fast if you are on a medication or have a medical condition without consulting your doctor.
- Don't fast if you are underweight.
- Children must not fast.
- Pregnant or nursing mothers must not fast.
- Don't fast if you have or have had an eating disorder.
- Fasting reduces food intake. It is imperative to eat nutrient rich food (the do's above) to compensate for the reduced quantity. Fasting on the Standard American Diet is not recommended as the standard diet is already deficient in macronutrients.

- Don't fast for much more than 24 hours. The human body has sufficient glucose reserves stored for a one day fast. During the fast, insulin levels drop and glucose is released from the liver to keep the brain nourished. As the fast progresses, the insulin level continues to drop encouraging the body to use our stored fat reserves. The body transitions into ketosis where the majority of our energy needs is supplied by fat and not glucose; however, the brain still needs glucose. After about 24 hours, the liver glucose reserves are running low and the body is starting to convert protein (muscle) into glucose causing muscle mass loss at rate of round 1 lb per day. This is starvation[17].

Bottom line is this: If you periodically fast for up to 24 hours, good things happen. You lose body fat without losing muscle, lower your cholesterol, and improve your insulin sensitivity. What happens if one periodically fasts for longer, say for 48 hours or 72 hours, which causes body to enter into starvation mode and loose lean body mass? We don't know as there are no studies on periodic starvation. Until such a study is done, it is better to stick to 24 hour or shorter fasts.

PROTEIN ON A PLANT-BASED DIET

Most nutrition guidelines recommend a fairly modest protein intake. The DRI (Dietary Reference Intake) is 0.8 grams of protein per kilogram of body weight, or 0.36 grams per pound. This amounts to 56 grams per day for the average sedentary man and 46 grams per day for the average sedentary woman. Higher amounts are not helpful and may be harmful. In terms of energy, the optimal protein intake is about 2.2 g protein for every 100 kcal of food eaten.

As Table 2 shows, meat has a high protein density (6-16 g/100 kcal depending on fat content), which is way above our target of 2.2 g/100 kcal. If you eat meat every day, you are almost guaranteed to get too much protein.

Surprisingly many people, who have lived eating meat, are worried about sufficient protein intake on a plant-based diet. This worry is largely misplaced. As Table 2 shows, vegetables contain significant amounts of protein. Per calorie basis, the protein content of broccoli, spinach, and mushrooms is comparable to meat. In fact, by eating just vegetables, one can exceed the recommended protein intake by a large margin; however, studies show that excess plant-based protein is not harmful and a high-plant protein diet may prolong life.

There are a two caveats: 1.) Plants are not energy dense and one needs to eat a lots of them to get both the required calories and protein. A diet high in refined carbohydrates and fats provides the needed calories but not the protein. 2.) Unlike meat, most plants do not contain all different protein types and one needs to eat different types of plants to obtain complete set of proteins. For example, legumes and grains combined provide complete protein. In addition, a few plants such as soy, quinoa, hemp seeds, or buckwheat are sources of complete proteins.

Bottom line is that by eating a variety of plant-based foods, sufficient protein intake is trivially easy to achieve. If one also eats significant amount animal products, too much protein becomes a concern.

TABLE 2.
PROTEIN DENSITY OF SELECTED FOODS

FOOD ITEM	G OF PROTEIN PER 100 KCAL
SPINACH	20
MEAT	6 - 16
TOFU	11
FISH	10
BROCCOLI	10
MUSHROOMS	7.5
BLACK BEANS	7
KALE	5
CARROTS	3
TARGET	2.2
NUTS	2
BLUEBERRIES	1.3
AVOCADO	1.2
BANANAS	1
APPLES	0

EVIDENCE ON SATURATED FATS

The role of saturated fats is a hotly debated topic. Most health organizations, including the American Heart Association and the World Health Organization (WHO), recommend reducing saturated fat intake but proponents of, for example, the Paleo diet challenge the mainstream guidelines. The proponents of saturated fats note that increase in fat intake can raise the HDL cholesterol.

Here is what we know:

- Replacing saturated fat with unsaturated fat improves cholesterol levels (p. 39)[11].
- Meals containing saturated fat have negative cardiovascular effect immediately after a meal (p. 50).
- Milk fat is associated with increased mortality (p. 37).
- Saturated fats reduce insulin sensitivity (p. 68).
- Plant-based diets that avoid all animal fats have the best record in treating and reversing coronary heart disease[12].

Based on the above, it is reasonable to conclude that avoiding saturated fats is a good idea especially as saturated fats do not have any demonstrable health benefits over unsaturated fats. If increased fat intake is desired to raise HDL cholesterol, unsaturated fats such as olive oil are a better choice as they raise HDL while also lowering LDL cholesterol. An even better option is to exercise more, which also raises HDL.

Some recent population studies, however, fail to demonstrate clear, causal links between saturated fat intake and increased mortality[10]. In fact, data indicates that a diet high in refined carbohydrates may be even more toxic to heart health than a diet high in saturated fats. This does not mean that saturated fats are healthy - it just means that fats are not a dietary monster in comparison to other unhealthy foods. If we choose to reduce saturated fat intake, we should substitute it with something healthier (the do's!) to benefit.

The Evidence Based Diet allows eating foods that contain saturated fats (for example meat) in moderation. Indigenous People who eat small amounts fat from animal products and exercise daily can maintain ideal cholesterol levels. It is possible to achieve the optimal cholesterol levels in modern settings too but it is not easy. To reach our cholesterol targets, we should make use of all the dietary tools available. This includes favoring unsaturated fats over saturated fats (olive oil over butter) and eating animal products in moderation.

Bottom line: If you achieve optimal cholesterol while eating saturated fats, your diet is working for you. If your cholesterol is hovering around 200 mg/dL (5.2 mmol/L), you should employ all tools available to lower it to optimal levels. This includes restricting saturated fat intake.

COMPARISON TO OTHER DIETS

Most diets are based on the idea of how we should eat. For example, vegans believe one should not eat animal products. Paleo dieters believe our genetics require eating like hunter gatherers. The Evidence Based Diet does not start with a fixed premise for the right diet. Due to this flexibility, the Evidence Based Diet is compatible with many popular diets including the vegan and Paleo diets.

Almost any diet is better than the Standard American Diet (SAD). A widely cited study comparing three diets - low-fat, Mediterranean, and low-carbohydrate - found that all resulted in a similar weight loss and small improvement in LDL cholesterol over a two-year period[9]. Unfortunately, none of the studied diets resulted in a sufficient improvement: The average BMI dropped from 31 kg/m^2 to 29-30 kg/m^2 and LDL cholesterol remained around 130 mg/dL (this with a quarter of study participants on cholesterol lowering medication!). This study is sometimes used as an evidence to show that a low-carbohydrate diet is as healthy as a low-fat diet but the conclusion misses the point. The results are simply not good enough and more drastic changes are needed.

In this section, the Evidence Based Diet is compared to other popular diets. I identify what the Evidence Based Diet has in common with these diets and how the diets can be improved using the Evidence Based Diet.

VEGAN DIET

In population studies, as a group, vegans are among the healthiest in modern society. Being vegan, however, is no guarantee of good health. It requires considerable effort to obtain all micro- and macronutrients from a purely plant-based diet. Plant foods are commonly not calorically dense and one needs to eat them in large volumes to satisfy even basic energy needs. As a consequence, it is all too easy to compensate by eating processed, energy-dense foods such as chips, bread, pasta, vegan cheese, fries, chocolate, cookies, and snack bars. This is obviously not compatible with the Evidence Based Diet which emphasizes consuming low-glycemic index and unrefined/unprocessed foods.

In addition, vegans can be deficient in vitamin B12, iron, calcium, zinc, and vitamin D. Taking supplements is a good insurance against deficiency. For B12, it is imperative.

Having said this, the plant-based vegan diet with adequate B12 supplementation is health promoting and compatible with the Evidence Based Diet.

PALEO DIET

The Paleo diet is based on the idea that our genetics are well suited for eating foods that were available 50,000 years ago. Accordingly, processed foods are avoided, as are grains and legumes (beans, peas, soybeans, peanuts, and tofu).

Evidence suggests that the hunter-gatherer diet, which includes small amounts of animal products and large amounts of fibrous vegetables, can achieve ideal cholesterol levels. Unfortunately, people eating the "modern Paleo diet" usually do not achieve the same cholesterol levels. A survey of Paleo recipes quickly shows why: meat is often the main ingredient in a Paleo meal. Not only is this bad for your heart but increases cancer risk and easily raises BMI.

A Paleo diet is compatible with the Evidence Based Diet if most calories are derived from plants and not from animal products. This is doable but harder than it needs to be: A Paleo diet does not allow all modern plant foods (grains and legumes) and one needs to eat even more vegetables to compensate which may become monotonous. Even then, fasting may be helpful in reaching optimal BMI and cholesterol levels.

LOW-CARB DIET

Low-carb diets such as the Atkins diet focus on controlling insulin levels to manage body weight. Refined carbohydrates are avoided as they raise insulin levels. The quality of carbohydrates, however, is important. Replacing refined carbohydrates with fat and animal protein may be an improvement over the Standard American Diet but it is not an optimal approach according to the Evidence Based Diet. Unprocessed carbohydrates in the form of plants (vegetables, legumes, fruits) or whole grains do not raise insulin any more than meat and they protect from cancer and diabetes.

Most versions of low-carb diets allow vegetables but restrict fruits and grains (even whole grains). This is an improvement over the Atkins diet but even these low-carb diets have a danger that is similar to the Paleo diet: by eliminating many plants from the diet, the animal products such as meat, milk, and cheese easily become a significant part of the diet. This raises the cholesterol levels, which increases the risk of heart disease.

A low-carb diet is compatible with the Evidence Based Diet if plants still form the majority of the calorie intake. A low-carb diet that is high in plant protein and plant-based fats improves health and life expectancy[23]. Good low-carb foods include avocado, broccoli, cauliflower, spinach, zucchini, green beans, kale, and tofu. In contrast, a low-carb diet high in animal protein and fats lowers life expectancy and is not compatible with the Evidence Based Diet.

KETOGENIC DIET

Ketogenic diet is an extreme version of the low-carb diet. The goal of the diet is to induce ketosis where energy is derived primarily from fats. The diet is characterized by very low carbohydrate, moderate protein, and high fat intake. To minimize carbohydrates, the diet is typically heavy on animal products such as meats, eggs, and dairy. Ketogenic diet has been used to treat epileptic patients that do not response drug treatments. More recently, ketogenic diet has been in vogue as a weight loss diet.

A ketogenic diet is difficult to follow. To induce and maintain ketosis, the carbohydrate intake has to be continuously very low. This is difficult. Even in clinical trials, less than 20% are able to maintain ketosis[16]. Side effects of the ketogenic diet include constipation (68%), headache (60%), muscle cramps (35%), diarrhea (23%), and general weakness (25%). Eating supplements is recommended as fat has no micronutrients.

Those who are able to follow a ketogenic diet report weight loss and improved blood glucose levels; however, the cholesterol levels are generally very high (LDL>130 mg/dL). We do not yet have sufficient information about the long-term effect of ketogenic diet on heart health to conclusively assess the effect of high cholesterol on ketosis. A study shows increased arterial wall stiffness which is an early marker of vascular damage[21]. However, a ketogenic diet based on olive oil might not show negative vascular effects[22]. In addition to the heart health, long-term concerns on ketogenic diet include kidney stones, increased cancer risk, and bone loss[24].

Since ketogenic diet severely limits fruit and vegetable consumption, it is not compatible with the Evidence Based Diet. This may change in the future when long-term studies on the risks and benefits of a ketogenic diet become available. Until then, it is safer to follow a more plant-based diet. If you do decide to experiment with ketogenic diet, the best approach may be to maximize the consumption of low-carb, plant-based foods. These include kale, avacodos, nuts, and seeds. For fat intake, it is good idea to emphasize unsaturated fats such as olive oil.

LOW-FAT DIET

A low-fat diet is inspired by the observation that saturated fats raise LDL cholesterol and hence increase heart disease risk. Low-fat diets, however, needlessly avoid all fats. Good fats (monounsaturated and polyunsaturated fats), when cosumed in moderation, lower LDL cholesterol levels and do not increase heart disease risk.

The biggest risk in low-fat diets is that many commercial low-fat foods are high in processed carbohydrates. If you follow a low-fat diet, I recommend focusing on avoiding saturated fats and eating whole plants instead. The Evidence Based Diet is low in saturated fats since it limits the use of animal products and replaces them with naturally low fat plant-based foods. Thus, the Evidence Based Diet is compatible with a low-fat diet while placing an emphasis on the quality of the carbohydrates (whole plants vs. refined carbohydrates).

CALORIE RESTRICTION

The calorie restriction diet was popularized by Dr. Walford who studied ways to extend the human lifespan[18]. In laboratory experiments on mouse and rats, the lifespan can be extended by to 50% when the animals are fed significantly less food than they would naturally eat. Moreover, the animals live healthier lives with a greatly reduced rate of age-related diseases such as cancer.

Longevity experiments with humans are not practical - it would take more than 60 years to obtain data from human experiments and the study would pose serious ethical dilemmas. Lacking the possibility to carry out human experiments, our primate relatives are the best option to study the effect of calorie restriction on aging. Inspired by the promising results from rodent studies, two calorie-restriction experiments with Rhesus monkeys were started in the 80s. Now, more than 30 years later, we have the first results[20].

The data from the primate experiments is both disappointing and encouraging: the maximum lifespan of primates is not increased by calorie restriction but diseases such as cancer and diabetes are greatly reduced. And the most encouraging result is that the disease-risk reduction is largely achieved by feeding the monkeys their recommended daily intake - no more and no less. In other words, we do not need to starve ourselves to get the most benefits of calorie restriction.

The Evidence Based Diet is compatible with a lite version of calorie restriction. By eating mostly plant-based foods, avoiding refined carbohydrates, and not overeating, the calorie intake is naturally reduced. For added measure, fasting is encouraged to lower BMI to the lower end of the normal range. However, the Evidence Based Diet does not advocate lowering our body mass below our natural baseline. We do not have sufficient evidence to show benefits and there are potential risks for such an extreme diet.

ADAPTING TO YOUR NEW DIET

Changing diet is demonstrably difficult. The majority of us want to eat healthy; yet, most of us continue to make bad dietary choices. The challenges are easy to understand when we consider that eating is more than just providing nutrition to our body. It is about the pleasure of eating, about our culture, memories, and the people we interact with. Some people may even be addicted to eating certain foods.

Improving eating habits is not easy and we cannot expect it to happen overnight. Instead, adopting a healthy diet is a process that builds on small successes. Viewed this way, a healthy diet is like learning a new skill. It takes time, effort, and persistence to make incremental changes. Over time, the changes add to meaningfully improved health outcomes.

Our goal is to optimize health based on the latest nutritional science. The data, however, is inconclusive. For example, we know that optimal cholesterol levels might be reached with a purely vegan diet. Or, we may achieve optimal cholesterol by continuing to eat some animal products but fasting for 24 hours 1-3 times per week. We do not have data to show which approach is better so the Evidence Based Diet allows you to decide which dietary tools to use based on your personal preferences.

The path to a healthy diet varies depending on the individuals and their life situations. The following ideas may be helpful in adapting to a healthier diet:

- Know your BMI, cholesterol, fasting glucose, and blood pressure numbers. This will tell you where you are and how changes in your diet can improve these values. Taking an active role in maintaining your health and seeing measurable improvements in health markers is an immensely satisfying and motivating experience.

- Recognize that the human palette is very adaptable. Is there a food that you could not live without? Chances are that if you did not eat it for 6 months, you wouldn't really miss it anymore. Conversely, you would learn to enjoy healthy foods by just eating more of them.
- Hunger is the best spice. For example, if you have eaten bacon and eggs for breakfast for decades, porridge with berries may not sound as appealing. A trick is to eat only when you are really hungry. For instance, eat a light dinner or skip it completely and the morning porridge will taste a lot better. If that is not enough, then fast for 24 hours and the porridge is going to be the best breakfast you have ever eaten!
- Be prepared to eat food in much larger quantities than you are used to. Plants are not energy dense foods and one needs to eat a lot more than on a diet based on animal products. It is good idea to have an easy access to healthy foods while adapting to a plant-based diet. Stock up so you are not tempted to eat something unhealthy.
- Stop eating all processed snacks and sweets immediately. Sugary snacks are unhealthy, but more importantly, sugary snacks alter taste bud preferences and create cravings for eating more snacks. It is impossible to enjoy a healthy salad if you are fantasizing of sugary snack bars. If you are used to eating sugary snacks, it may help to have alternative low-calorie vegetables such as carrots and cauliflower to nibble on.
- Don't have junk food around your house.
- Think of meat as a spice and not the main ingredient.
- Have meatless days where you do not consume any animal products. A meatless Monday is a great start to a more plant-based diet.
- Social aspects of eating can complicate the transition to a more plant-based diet. For example, it may be difficult to change family dinners where the family's favorite foods are usually served. Instead of changing the whole family's diet immediately, it may be helpful to first change the meals that don't involve the social element. Eating different breakfast foods or eating differently during a workplace lunch should not offend other family members. Change these meals first. Meanwhile, talk to your family about what you are doing and what you are trying to achieve. Chances are that your family members will be supportive. They may even be interested in improving their own diet too. When your family is ready, try new recipes together as a family or visit a vegan restaurant.

- It is easy to "veganize" some common foods. For example, tacos are great with beans, guacamole, salsa, corn, and lettuce. They also work well as family meals if some family members prefer to eat meat.
- Don't fall for vegan alternatives. Vegan bacon will only make you want to eat the real thing. Your goal should be to train your taste buds to enjoy the taste of healthy foods, not pale and processed imitation of your old foods.
- Don't preach about your diet. It's okay to be silently smug about eating well but that is as far as it should go. Food and nutrition are touchy topics and best to be avoided. Instead, try talking about religion, politics, or other safer topics.
- If anyone asks about your diet, have a simple answer that avoids ethical dilemmas. For example, replying that you are trying to lower your cholesterol should not offend anyone.
- Feel free to experiment with different approaches and new foods. Part of the fun in changing your diet is the discovery of new recipes and tastes. Web is full of amazing plant-based recipes.

EPILOGUE

This book started as a personal quest to improve health and minimize disease risks. Thus, the success for this book is not measured in sales but whether I could achieve a marked improvement in my health numbers. The answer is a definite yes. Table 3 below shows my numbers before and after adopting the Evidence Based Diet. The improvement is significant and comparable to or better than the best results from clinical trials.

TABLE 3. AUTHOR'S HEALTH MARKERS

MONTHS OF EVIDENCE BASED DIET	LDL [MG/DL] (MMOL/L)	TOTAL CHOLESTEROL [MG/DL] (MMOL/L)	FASTING GLUCOSE [MG/DL] (MMOL/L)	BMI [KG/M2
0	128 (3.3)	197 (5.1)	98 (5.4)	24.1
6	106 (2.7)	180 (4.7)	98 (5.4)	22.7
12	105 (2.7)	174 (4.5)	96 (5.3)	22.5
16	68 (1.8)	127 (3.3)	91 (5.1)	22.1
20	77 (2.0)	134 (3.5)	89 (4.9)	22.1

During the first year, I kept tweaking the diet to be more plant-based. I estimate that I was eating purely plant-based diet on approximately 70% of the days. On remaining days, about twice per week, I would also eat meat, fish, or dairy. This resulted in significant improvement in health markers. The cholesterol dropped to near optimal level of <180 mg/dL which corresponds to an increase of 3+ years in life expectancy. After the initial drop, however, the cholesterol levels seemed to stabilize above my targets. Between 6 and 12 month measurements, my LDL cholesterol remained virtually unchanged and above 100 mg/dL.

After 12 months, I increased the number of plant days further to about 85% of all days, eliminated almost all meat and dairy, and ate fish about once a week. In addition, I ate a small number of eggs (1-2 eggs per week) and meat one to two times per month. Due to business trips, I did not follow this diet all the time but the results were still amazing: The total cholesterol dropped to 127 mg/dL (-36% from baseline) and LDL cholesterol dropped to 68 mg/dL (-47% from baseline). At these levels, cardiovascular disease progression is halted or even reversed. In addition, fasting glucose improved by 7%, my vitamin D and calcium levels are excellent, homocysteine is 10.2 µmol/L, and the apo B/A-I ratio is below 0.60. I am no longer worried about heart disease.

After some experimenting, here is my current diet:

- Apart from the fish once per week and few eggs, I do not consume any animal products. No milk, cheese, or butter.
- No processed carbohydrates. This means for example no bread, pasta, candy, or soda.
- For calcium, I eat greens and drink fortified non-dairy milks.
- I eat a daily multivitamin that is formulated for vegans. The multivitamin is an insurance that I am not deficient in iron, zinc, or calcium which are common concerns on a plant-based diet.
- I take weekly vitamin D and B12 supplements as the multivitamin does not provide sufficient dose of these two critical vitamins. The choice of taking weekly supplement is simply due to a convenient weekly dose being available.
- Small handful of nuts every day.
- For lunch, I usually eat either a green smoothie (greens, frozen berries, oats, fruits, and flax seeds) or raw vegetables, hummus, and nuts or a salad.
- I experimented with different fasting regimens and found that time-restricted eating works best for me. I usually do not eat breakfast. This extends the overnight fast until lunch. I also try not to eat after dinner so that all eating happens in a 6-to-8 hour window between noon and dinner.

- I don't practice calorie restriction but I try to maintain BMI in the lower end of the normal range. In addition to skipping breakfast, I try to stop eating when I am almost full. This, combined with plant-based diet, has been enough to reduce my BMI to the low 20s.
- If my body weight starts to increase, I do one day fast. This seems to reset my portion size so that I do not overeat. I have found that a fast day once a month is sufficient for me to prevent the weight gain.

I find it notable that I reached the optimal cholesterol numbers while still consuming some animal products (mainly fish and eggs). This confirms that being purely vegan is not the only option to maintain perfect hearth health. Focusing on quality foods, eating mostly plant-based foods, and not eating junk may be the key to healthy diet.

Yet, I cannot fully explain the big improvement between 12-month and 16-month measurements. I speculate the human body response is nonlinear as it nears the optimal diet and BMI. Near optimum, small changes in diet can have a big effect. As most diet studies are carried out on the Standard American Diet and higher BMI as the baseline, there is little evidence to support this hypothesis; however, the bottom line is that the Evidence Based Diet works.

Looking back, I am amazed how easy it was to lower the cholesterol to hunter-gatherer levels. Yes, it did require big, and at times even painful, changes but I am still eating regular grocery store foods including vegetables, legumes, fruits, fish, eggs, and very little meat. There are diets that are much more extreme than this. But maybe the Evidence Based Diet is not for everyone: I discussed the diet with my doctor who was very impressed with my cholesterol results (he called them a miracle). After listening for a few minutes, he said that he could not do it. More than likely, he also won't recommend a plant-based diet to his other patients, even if the evidence shows major health benefits. It is no wonder that there is so much confusion about diets as even many health professionals are captive to their unhealthy eating habits.

While improvement in health numbers was my primary goal in developing the Evidence Based Diet, I gained a surprising but equally important secondary benefit: I now feel healthier. I have less seasonal allergies and digestive problems, my skin rashes have disappeared, and feel less tired and more energetic. I did not expect this. The feeling of wellbeing is a hard thing to quantify, and it is therefore not mentioned in the scientific publications cited in this book. Yet, everyone I have talked to, who has dismissed the Standard American Diet (SAD) to eat something healthier, has confirmed that they also feel better. If you are yet to experience this, I urge you to try out how you will feel on a plant-based diet. (If you don't notice improvement, you can always go back.)

I fully understand that my personal results do not meet the criteria for a clinical study and may not be representative of what others will achieve with a similar diet. Our bodies are different and may respond differently to changes in our diet. Nevertheless, I hope that the evidence in this book and my personal experience inspire you to experiment with, and improve, your diet.

Diet and nutritional advice is constantly evolving and this book will evolve with the latest scientific research. Please follow me on twitter @DietEvidence to keep on top of latest news, ask questions, or to share your success story. I would love to hear from you!

Ville Kaajakari, PhD

REFERENCES

[1] D. M. Lloyd-Jones, E. P. Leip, M. G. Larson, R. B. d'Agostino, A. Beiser, P. W. F. Wilson, P. A. Wolf, and D. Levy, "Prediction of lifetime risk for cardiovascular disease by risk factor burden at 50 years of age," Circulation 113, No. 6 (2006): 791-798.

[2] B. Armstrong, and R. Doll, "Environmental factors and cancer incidence and mortality in different countries, with special reference to dietary practices," International Journal of Cancer 15, No. 4 (1975): 617-631.

[3] A. G. Shaper and K. W. Jones, "Serum-cholesterol, diet, and coronary heart-disease in Africans and Asians in Uganda," The Lancet 274 (1959): 534-537.

[4] B. S. Lennerz, D. C. Alsop, L. M. Holsen, E. Stern, R. Rojas, C. B. Ebbeling, J. M. Goldstein, and D. S. Ludwig, "Effects of dietary glycemic index on brain regions related to reward and craving in men," The American Journal of Clinical Nutrition 98, No. 3 (2013): 641-647.

[5] D. J. Jenkins, T. H. Nguyen, C. W. Kendall, D. A. Faulkner, B. Bashyam, I. J. Kim, C. Ireland, D. Patel, E. Vidgen, A. R. Josse, and H. D. Sesso, "The effect of strawberries in a cholesterol-lowering dietary portfolio," Metabolism-Clinical and Experimental 57, No. 12 (2008): 1636-1644.

[6] D. L. Everett, Don't sleep, there are snakes: Life and language in the Amazonian jungle, Profile Books, 2009.

[7] R. Antoni, K. L. Johnston, A. Collins, and M. Robertson, "Intermittent versus continuous energy restriction: differential effects on postprandial glucose and lipid metabolism following matched weight-loss in overweight/obese subjects," British Journal of Nutrition 119, No. 5 (2018): 507-516.

[8] *D. Hyson, J. C. Rutledge, and L. Berglund, "Postprandial lipemia and cardiovascular disease," Current Atherosclerosis Reports 5 No. 6 (2003): 437-444.*

[9] *I. Shai, D. Schwarzfuchs, Y. Henkin, D. R. Shahar, S. Witkow, I. Greenberg, R. Golan, D. Fraser, A. Bolotin, H. Vardi, and O. Tangi-Rozental, "Weight loss with a low-carbohydrate, Mediterranean, or low-fat diet," New England Journal of Medicine 359 No. 3 (2008): 229-241.*

[10] *M. Dehghan, A. Mente, X. Zhang, S. Swaminathan, W. Li, V. Mohan, R. Iqbal, R. Kumar, E. Wentzel-Viljoen, A. Rosengren, and L. I.Amma, "Associations of fats and carbohydrate intake with cardiovascular disease and mortality in 18 countries from five continents (PURE): a prospective cohort study," The Lancet 390 (2017):2050-2062.*

[11] *L. Hodson, C. M. Skeaff, and W. A. Chisholm, "The effect of replacing dietary saturated fat with polyunsaturated or monounsaturated fat on plasma lipids in free-living young adults," European journal of clinical nutrition 55, No. 10 (2001):908-915.*

[12] *C. B. Esselstyn, "A plant-based diet and coronary artery disease: a mandate for effective therapy," Journal of Geriatric Cardiology 14, No. 5 (2017): 317-320.*

[13] *World Cancer Research Fund International, www.wcrf.org*

[14] *D. J Jenkins, C. W. Kendall, A. Marchie, D. A. Faulkner, J. M. Wong, R. de Souza, A. Emam, T. L. Parker, E. Vidgen, E. A. Trautwein, and K. G. Lapsley, "Direct comparison of a dietary portfolio of cholesterol-lowering foods with a statin in hypercholesterolemic participants," The American Journal of Clinical Nutrition 81, No. 2 (2005:) pp.380-387.*

[15] *R. W. Allen, Robert, E. Schwartzman, W. L. Baker, C. I. Coleman, and O. J. Phung, "Cinnamon use in type 2 diabetes: an updated systematic review and meta-analysis," The Annals of Family Medicine 11, No. 5 (2013): 452-459.*

[16] *W. S. Yancy, M. K. Olsen, J. R. Guyton, R. P. Bakst, and E. C. Westman, "A low-carbohydrate, ketogenic diet versus a low-fat diet to treat obesity and hyperlipidemia: a randomized, controlled trial," Annals of Internal Medicine 140, No. 10 (2004): 769-777.*

[17] *M. Elia, R. J. Stubbs, and C. J. K. Henry. "Differences in fat, carbohydrate, and protein metabolism between lean and obese subjects undergoing total starvation." Obesity Research 7, No. 6 (1999): 597-604.*

[18] *R. L. Walford, 120 year diet plan, Simon and Schuster, 1986.*

[19] J. A. Mattison, R. J. Colman, T. M. Beasley, D. B. Allison, J. W. Kemnitz, G. S. Roth, D. K. Ingram, R. Weindruch, R. De Cabo, and R. M. Anderson, "Caloric restriction improves health and survival of rhesus monkeys," Nature Communications 8, (2017): 14063.

[20] W. März, M. E. Kleber, H. Scharnagl, T. Speer, S. Zewinger, A. Ritsch, K. G. Parhofer, A. von Eckardstein, U. Landmesser, and U. Laufs, "HDL cholesterol: reappraisal of its clinical relevance," Clinical Research in Cardiology 106, No. 9 (2017): 663-675.

[21] C. Giangennaro, F. Natale, A. Torino, R. Capasso, A. D'Aniello, E. Pironti, E. Santoro, R. Calabró, and A. Verrotti, "The impact of the ketogenic diet on arterial morphology and endothelial function in children and young adults with epilepsy: A caseâ "control study," Seizure 23, No. 4 (2014): 260-265.

[22] Ö. Rahmi, O. Güzel, M. Küşük, C. Karadeniz, N. Katipoglu, Ü. Yılmaz, M. M. Yılmazer, and T. Meşe, "The effect of the ketogenic diet on the vascular structure and functions in children with intractable epilepsy," Pediatric neurology 56 (2016): 30-34.

[23] S. B. Seidelmann, B. Claggett, S. Cheng, M. Henglin, A. Shah, L. M. Steffen, A. R. Folsom, E. B. Rimm, W. C. Willett, and S. D. Solomon, "Dietary carbohydrate intake and mortality: a prospective cohort study and meta-analysis,"The Lancet Public Health 3, No. 9 (2018): e419-e428.

[24] A. G. C. Bergqvist, J. I. Schall, V. A. Stallings, and B. S. Zemel, "Progressive bone mineral content loss in children with intractable epilepsy treated with the ketogenic diet,"The American Journal of Clinical Nutrition 88, No. 6 (2008): 1678-1684.

Made in United States
North Haven, CT
10 November 2026

22095609R00083